STUDY GUIDE FOR

Nursing Research
principles and methods

Fourth edition

STUDY GUIDE FOR

Nursing Research
principles and methods

Fourth edition

Denise F. Polit, Ph.D.

President
Humanalysis, Inc.
Saratoga Springs, New York

Bernadette P. Hungler, R.N., Ph.D.

Associate Professor
Boston College School of Nursing
Chestnut Hill, Massachusetts

J. B. Lippincott Company
Philadelphia
New York   London   Hagerstown

Acquisition Editor: David Carroll
Coordinating Editorial Assistant: Amy Stonehouse
Production Supervisor: Susan Clarey
Production: Till & Till, Inc.
Compositor: The Composing Room of Michigan, Inc.
Printer/Binder: R.R. Donnelley & Sons

Any procedure or practice described in this book should be applied
by the health-care practitioner under appropriate supervision in
accordance with professional standards of care used with regard to
the unique circumstances that apply in each practice situation. Care
has been taken to confirm the accuracy of information presented and
to describe generally accepted practices. However, the authors,
editors and publisher cannot accept any responsibility for errors or
omissions or for consequences from application of the information in
this book and make no warranty, express or implied, with respect to
the contents of the book.

Every effort has been made to ensure drug selections and dosages are
in accordance with current recommendations and practice. Because of
ongoing research, changes in government regulations, and the
constant flow of information on drug therapy, reactions, and
interactions, the reader is cautioned to check the package insert
for each drug for indications, dosages, warnings, and precautions,
particularly if the drug is new or infrequently used.

Preface

This Study Guide has been prepared to complement the fourth edition of *Nursing Research: Principles and Methods*. The guide provides opportunities to reinforce the acquisition of basic research skills through systematic learning exercises. The book is also intended to help bridge the gap between the passive reading of complex, abstract materials and active participation in the development of research skills through concrete examples and study suggestions.

As in the case of the textbook, this Study Guide was developed on the premise that research examples are a critical component of the learning process. The inclusion of actual and fictitious research examples is designed to instruct (i.e., facilitate the absorption of research concepts); motivate (i.e., encourage curiosity and an interest in acquiring research skills); and stimulate (i.e., suggest topics that might be pursued further by nurse researchers and practicing nurses interested in the utilization of research findings).

The Study Guide consists of 30 chapters—one chapter corresponding to every chapter in the textbook. Each of the 30 chapters (except for one) consists of five sections:

- *Matching Exercises.* Terms and concepts presented in the textbook are reinforced by having students perform a matching routine that often involves matching the concrete (e.g., actual hypotheses) with the abstract (e.g., type of hypotheses).

- *Completion Exercises.* Sentences are presented in which the student must fill in a missing word or phrase corresponding to important ideas presented in the textbook.

- *Study Questions.* Each chapter contains two to five short individual exercises relevant to the materials in the textbook, including the preparation of definitions of terms.

- *Application Exercises.* These exercises, geared primarily to the consumers of nursing research, involve opportunities to critique various aspects of a study. Each chapter contains both fictitious research examples and suggestions for one or more actual research examples, which students are asked to evaluate according to a dimension emphasized in the corresponding chapter of the textbook. The critique is facilitated by a series of guiding questions, which should also serve to stimulate class discussion.

- *Special Projects.* This section, geared primarily to the producers of nursing research, offers suggestions for fairly large projects in which, in many cases, an entire classroom could collaborate.

Like the textbook, this Study Guide is expected to find application at both the undergraduate and graduate levels, and may be of heuristic value to practicing nurses as well.

Contents

Part V: The Analysis of Research Data

Part VI: Communication in the Research Process

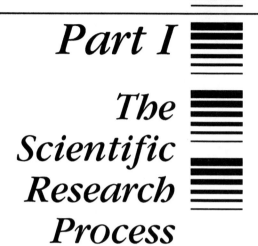

Part I

The Scientific Research Process

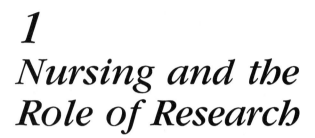

1
Nursing and the
Role of Research

A. Matching Exercises

Match each of the activities in Set B with one of the time frames in Set A. Indicate the letter corresponding to the appropriate response next to each entry in Set B.

SET A
a. Pre-1950s
b. 1950s
c. 1960s
d. 1970s
e. 1980s to present

SET B	RESPONSE
1. Nursing research focused on nurses themselves	_____
2. Increased research focus on clinical problems	_____
3. Establishment of the National Center for Nursing Research at the National Institutes of Health	_____
4. Creation of the professional journal *Research in Nursing and Health*	_____
5. First nursing research study was conducted	_____
6. Creation of the professional journal *Nursing Research*	_____

  7. Increased interest in theoretical bases for conducting nursing research _____

  8. Both ANA and NLN make recommendations regarding the research preparation of nurses _____

  9. Growing interest in in-depth, process-oriented studies _____

  10. Establishment of a nursing archive at Boston University _____

  11. Nursing unit focusing on research established at Walter Reed _____

  12. Winslow–Goldmark report focusing on nursing education released _____

B. Completion Exercises

Write the words or phrases that correctly complete the sentences below.

  1. Research in nursing began with _____

  _____

  2. During the early years, the majority of nursing studies focused on _____

  _____

  3. The school of nursing at Yale came into being as a result of the _____

  _____ investigation.

  4. The rapid acceleration of nursing research began in the _____

  _____

  5. The _____ ,

  created by the American Nurses' Association, was founded for the promotion of

  nursing research.

  6. The future direction of nursing research is likely to involve a continuing focus on

  _____

C. Study Questions

  1. Define the following terms. Compare your definition with the definition in Chapter 1 or in the glossary.

     a. Producer of nursing research: _____

_____

_____

b. Consumer of nursing research: _____

_____

_____

c. Accountability: _____

_____

_____

d. The Winslow–Goldmark report: _____

_____

_____

e. National Center for Nursing Research: _____

_____

_____

f. WICHEN: _____

_____

_____

2. Why is it important for nurses who will never conduct their own research to understand scientific methods?

3. What are some potential consequences to the profession of nursing if nurses stopped conducting their own research?

4. Provide an example of how research might play a role in each of the following phases associated with the Standards for Nursing Practice.

   a. Assessment phase: _____

   _____

   _____

    b. Diagnosis phase: _____

    _____

    _____

    c. Planning phase: _____

    _____

    _____

    d. Intervention phase: _____

    _____

    _____

    e. Evaluation phase: _____

    _____

    _____

5. Many students have concerns about courses on research methods. Complete the following sentences, expressing as honestly as possible your own feelings about research, and discuss your concerns with your class.

    a. I (am/am not) looking forward to this class on nursing research because:

    _____

    _____

    b. I think that I would like a course in nursing research methods better if:

    _____

    _____

    c. I think a class in nursing research (will/will not) improve my effectiveness as a nurse because: _____

    _____

    _____

6. What are some of the current changes occurring in the health-care delivery system and how could these changes influence nursing research?

2
The Scientific Approach

A. *Matching Exercises*

Match each of the research questions in Set B with one of the purposes for conducting research in Set A. Indicate the letter corresponding to the appropriate response next to each entry in Set B.

SET A
a. Description
b. Exploration
c. Explanation
d. Prediction/control

SET B   **RESPONSE**

1. What is the nature of the emotional experience of loneliness among the institutionalized elderly?   _____

2. What factors predict the use of contraceptives at first intercourse among teenage women?   _____

3. What percentage of women fail to receive prenatal care during the first trimester of a pregnancy?   _____

4. What are the underlying causes of burnout among RNs working in intensive care units?   _____

5. What is the process by which terminally ill patients take leave of their families and close friends?   _____

7

6. What types of characteristics are related to a woman's decision to return to work within six weeks postpartum? _____

7. Does vestibular stimulation affect the duration of quiet sleep among preterm infants? _____

8. Why are teenage mothers less likely to breastfeed their infants than older mothers? _____

B. Completion Exercises

Write the words or phrases that correctly complete the sentences below.

1. The approach to human knowledge that uses systematic, controlled procedures is known as the _____

_____

2. The process of developing generalizations from specific observations is referred to as _____

_____ reasoning.

3. The scientific assumption that all phenomena have antecedent causes is called

_____

4. The most ingrained source of knowledge, and the one that is the most difficult to challenge, is _____

_____

5. The characteristic of the scientific approach that enables researchers to rule out competing explanations is _____

_____

6. Since scientific inquiry is not concerned with isolated phenomena, a key characteristic of the scientific method is _____

_____

7. Of the various purposes of scientific inquiry, the one that epitomizes its spirit is

_____

8. The type of research that involves the systematic collection and analysis of controlled, numerical information is known as _____

9. The type of research that involves the systematic collection and analysis of subjective, narrative materials is known as _____

10. The scientific approach has as its philosophical underpinnings a school of thought known as _____

C. Study Questions

1. Define the following terms. Compare your definition with the definition in Chapter 2 or in the glossary.

   a. Empiricism: _____

   _____

   _____

   b. Deductive reasoning: _____

   _____

   _____

   c. Authority as a source of knowledge: _____

   _____

   _____

   d. Applied research: _____

   _____

   _____

   e. Basic research: _____

   _____

   _____

   f. Assumption: _____

   _____

   _____

g. Phenomenology: _____

_____

_____

2. Below are several research problems. For each, indicate whether you think it is *primarily* an applied or basic research question.

RESEARCH PROBLEM	TYPE
a. Does movement tempo affect perception of the passage of time?	_____
b. Does follow-up by nurses improve patients' compliance with their medication regimen?	_____
c. Does the ingestion of cranberry juice reduce urinary tract infections?	_____
d. Is sweat gland activity related to ACTH levels?	_____
e. Is pain perception associated with a person's locus of control (an aspect of personality)?	_____
f. Does the type of nursing curriculum affect attrition rates in schools of nursing?	_____
g. Does nicotine affect postural muscle tremor?	_____
h. Does the nurse/patient ratio affect nurses' job satisfaction?	_____

3. Below are descriptions of several research problems. Indicate whether you think the problem is best suited to a qualitative or quantitative approach, and indicate why you think this is so.
   a. What is the decision-making process of AIDS patients seeking treatment?

   b. What effect does room temperature have on the colonization rate of bacteria in urinary catheters?

   c. What are the sources of stress among nursing home residents?

   d. Does therapeutic touch affect the vital signs of hospitalized patients?

4. What are some of the limitations of quantitative research? What are some of the limitations of qualitative research? Which approach seems best suited to address problems in which you might be interested? Why is that?

D. Application Exercises

Duffy (1990)* studied the effect of the wording of communications on encouraging the elderly to come forward for a flu vaccination. All members of a senior citizens center in a mid-sized community (a total of 500 elderly men and women) were sent a letter advising them that a flu epidemic was anticipated that season and that the elderly were especially likely to benefit from an immunization. Half of the members were sent a letter stressing the benefits of getting a flu shot. The other half of the members were sent a letter stressing the potential dangers of *not* getting a flu shot. To avoid any biases, a "lottery" type system was used to determine who got which letter. All of the elderly were advised that free immunizations would be available at a community health clinic over a one-week period and that free transportation would also be made available to them. Duffy monitored the rates of coming forward for a flu shot among the two groups of elderly to assess whether one approach of encouragement was more persuasive than the other.

1. Consider the aspects of this study vis-à-vis the issues discussed in this chapter. To assist you in your review, here are some guiding questions.

   a. Do the features of this study correspond to the characteristics of the scientific approach? To what extent are the characteristics of order, control, empiricism, generalization, and theory represented in this example?

   b. How would you characterize the purpose of this study? Is its major aim description, exploration, explanation, prediction, or control? Is there more than one purpose? Would you say this study is an example of basic or applied research?

   c. The main purpose of the study is to examine the relationship between the type of communcation and the preventive health behavior of the elderly. Review the various "limitations of the scientific method" discussed in Chapter 2 and consider whether and how each applies to the study under consideration.

   d. In this study, would it be more appropriate to collect and analyze qualitative or quantitative information? Why do you think this is so?

2. Below are several suggested research articles. Skim one or more of these articles and respond to questions a to d from Question D.1 in terms of an actual research study:

   • Mattson, S. (1990). Coping and developmental maturity of R.N. Baccalaureate students. *Western Journal of Nursing Research, 12,* 514–524.

   • Nettles-Carlson, B., *et al.* (1988). Effectiveness of teaching breast self-examination during office visits. *Research in Nursing and Health, 11,* 41–50.

*The example is fictitious.

- Solheim, K. and Spellacy, C. (1988). Sibling visitation: Effects on newborn infection rates. *Journal of Obstetric, Gynecologic, and Neonatal Nursing, 17*, 43–48.

E. Special Projects

1. Consider the following research statement:

    The purpose of this study is to understand why nurses are or are not satisfied with their jobs.

    The basic purpose of this study as stated is descriptive. Alter the statement in such a way as to design a study whose essential purpose is exploration; explanation; prediction; and control.

2. Think of the last "fact" you learned with respect to clinical nursing practice. Try to discover the ultimate source of this information. Was it tradition ("This is the way it's always been done")? Authority ("Dr. So-and-so said so")? Logical reasoning ("This has been inferred from previous observations")? Or scientific method ("An empirical investigation discovered this to be the case")?

3
Ethics and
Scientific Research

A. Matching Exercises

Match each of the descriptions in Set B with one of the procedures used to safeguard human subjects from Set A. Indicate the letter corresponding to the appropriate response next to each entry in Set B.

SET A
a. Freedom from harm or exploitation
b. Informed consent
c. Anonymity
d. Confidentiality

SET B   **RESPONSE**

1. A questionnaire distributed by mail bears an ID number in one corner. Respondents are assured their responses will not be individually divulged.   _____

2. Hospitalized children included in a study, and their parents, are told the aims and procedures of the research. Parents are asked to sign an authorization.   _____

3. Respondents in a questionnaire study in which the same respondents will be questioned twice are asked to place their own four-digit ID on the questionnaire and to memorize the ID number. Respondents are assured their answers will remain private. _____

4. Women who recently had a mastectomy are studied in terms of psychological sequelae. In the interview, sensitive questions are carefully worded. After the interview, debriefing with the respondent determines the need for psychological support. _____

5. Women interviewed in the above study (number 4) are told that the information they provide will not be individually divulged. _____

6. Subjects who volunteered for an experimental treatment for AIDS are warned of potential side effects and are asked to sign a waiver. _____

7. After determining that a new intervention resulted in discomfort to subjects, the researcher discontinued the study. _____

8. Unmarked questionnaires are distributed to a class of nursing students. The instructions indicate that the responses will not be individually divulged. _____

9. The researcher assures subjects that they will be interviewed as part of the study at a single point in time, and adheres to this promise. _____

10. A questionnaire distributed to a sample of nursing students includes a statement indicating that completion and submission of the questionnaire will be construed as voluntary participation in a study, as fully described in an accompanying letter. _____

B. Completion Exercises

Write the words or phrases that correctly complete the sentences below.

1. Ethical _____ arise when the rights of subjects and the demands of science are put into direct conflict.

2. One of the first internationally recognized efforts to establish ethical standards was the _____

3. The National Commission for the Protection of Human Subjects of Biomedical and Behavioral Research issued a well-known set of guidelines known as the

_____

4. The most straightforward ethical precept is the protection of subjects from

_____

5. Risks that are no greater than those ordinarily encountered in daily life are referred to as _____

_____

6. The right to _____
means that prospective subjects have the right to voluntarily decide whether or not to participate in a study, without risk of penalty.

7. The researcher adheres to the principle of _____

_____

by fully describing to subjects the nature of the study and the likely risks and benefits of participation.

8. When the researcher cannot link research information to the person who provided it, the condition known as _____

_____

has prevailed.

9. Special procedures are often required to safeguard the rights of _____

_____

subjects.

10. Committees established in institutions to review proposed research procedures with respect to their adherence to ethical guidelines are often called IRBs, or

_____

C. Study Questions

1. Define the following terms. Compare your definition with the definition in Chapter 3 or in the glossary.

   a. Human subjects: _____

   _____

   _____

b. Code of ethics: _____

_____

_____

c. Beneficence: _____

_____

_____

d. Debriefing: _____

_____

_____

e. Risk–benefit ratio: _____

_____

_____

f. Coercion: _____

_____

_____

g. Subject stipends: _____

_____

_____

h. Covert data collection: _____

_____

_____

i. Deception: _____

_____

_____

j. Confidentiality: _____

_____

_____

k. Informed consent: _____

_____

1. Expedited review: _____

_____

2. Below are descriptions of several research studies. Suggest some ethical dilemmas that are likely to emerge for each.

   a. A study of coping behaviors among rape victims

   _____

   b. An unobtrusive observational study of fathers' behaviors in the delivery room

   _____

   c. An interview study of the antecedents of heroin addiction

   _____

   d. A study of dependence among mentally retarded children

   _____

   e. An investigation of the verbal interactions among schizophrenic patients

   _____

   f. A study of the effects of a new drug on human subjects

   _____

3. Skim the article describing the study by Zimmerman *et al.* (1988) entitled "Effects of music in patients who had chronic cancer pain" (*Western Journal of Nursing Research, 11,* 298–309). Draft an informed consent form for this study.

   _____

   _____

4. At the beginning of Chapter 3 in the textbook, two unethical studies were described (the study of syphilis among black men and the study in which live cancer cells were injected in elderly patients). Identify which ethical principles were transgressed in these studies.

D. Application Exercises

Brenenstuhl (1991)* investigated the behavior of nursing students in crisis or emergency situations. The investigator was interested in comparing the behaviors of students from B.S. versus diploma programs to determine the adequacy of the preparation given to students in handling emergencies. Fifty students from both types of programs volunteered to participate in the study. The investigator wanted to observe reactions to crises as they might occur naturally, so the participants were not told the exact nature of the study. Each student was instructed to perform a simple task, purportedly to investigate reaction time. A second person, who was described as another participant but who in fact was a confederate of the investigator, simulated an epileptic seizure during the "experiment." An assistant to the investigator, who was unaware of the purpose of the study and who did not know the educational background of the subjects, observed the timeliness and appropriateness of the students' responses through a one-way mirror. Subjects were not required to fill out forms in which their identities were divulged. Immediately following participation, subjects were debriefed as to the true nature of the study.

1. Consider the aspects of this study vis-à-vis the issues discussed in this chapter. To assist you in your review, here are some guiding questions.

   a. Were the subjects in this study at risk of physical or psychological harm? Were they at risk of exploitation?

   b. Did the subjects in the study derive any benefits from their participation? Did the nursing community or society at large benefit? How would you assess the risk/benefit ratio?

   c. Were the subjects' rights to self-determination violated? Was there any coercion involved? Was full disclosure made to subjects prior to participation? Was informed consent given to subjects and documented?

   d. Were subjects treated fairly? Was their right to privacy protected?

   e. What ethical dilemmas does this study present? How, if at all, can the dilemmas be resolved? To what extent *were* they resolved?

---

*This study is fictitious.

    f. What type of human subjects review would be appropriate for a study such as the one described?

2. Read one or more of the articles listed in Table 3.2 of the textbook. Respond to questions a to f from Question D.1 above in terms of these actual research studies.

E. Special Projects

1. Prepare a brief summary of a hypothetical study in which there would be at least three major benefits to subjects participating in the study.
2. Prepare a brief summary of a hypothetical study in which the costs and benefits were both high. When the costs and benefits are essentially balanced, how should the researcher decide whether or not to proceed?

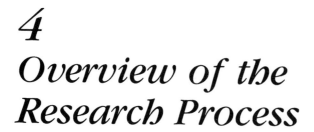

4
Overview of the Research Process

A. *Matching Exercises*

EXERCISE 1
Match each of the terms in Set B with one (or more) of the terms in Set A. Indicate the letter corresponding to your response next to each item in Set B.

SET A
a. Categorical variable
b. Continuous variable
c. Active variable
d. Attribute variable
e. Constant

SET B   **RESPONSE**

1. Employment status (working/not working)   _____
2. Dosage of a new drug   _____
3. Pi (π) (to calculate area of a circle)   _____
4. Number of times hospitalized   _____
5. Method of teaching patients (structured versus unstructured)   _____
6. Blood type   _____
7. pH level of urine   _____
8. Pulse rate of a deceased person   _____

9. Membership in a nursing union   _____
10. Birthweight of an infant   _____
11. Presence or absence of decubiti   _____
12. Degree of empathy in nurses   _____

EXERCISE 2

SET A
a. Independent variable
b. Dependent variable
c. Either/both

SET B	**RESPONSE**
1. The variable that is the presumed effect	_____
2. The variable that is dichotomous	_____
3. The variable that is the main outcome of interest in the study	_____
4. The variable that is the presumed cause	_____
5. The variable referred to as the criterion variable	_____
6. The variable that is an attribute	_____
7. The variable "length of stay in hospital"	_____
8. The variable that requires an operational definition	_____

B. Completion Exercises

Write the words or phrases that correctly complete the sentences below.

1. A small-scale trial run of a research study is referred to as a(n) _____

   _____

2. The total aggregate of units that a researcher is interested in is known as the

   _____

3. When a researcher carefully specifies the steps that must be taken to measure the

   concepts of interest, she or he develops _____

   _____

4. The variable that the researcher wants to understand, explain, or predict is known

   as the _____ or _____
   variable.

5. The two basic categories of sampling are referred to as _____

   _____ and _____
   sampling.

6. If a researcher studied the effect of a scheduling assignment on nurses' morale, scheduling assignment would be referred to as the _____ variable.

7. The pieces of information obtained in the course of a study are collectively known as the _____

   _____

8. The abstract qualities in which a researcher is interested are referred to in scientific parlance as _____

   or _____

9. The variable presumed to *cause* changes in some other variable is the _____

   _____

10. The researcher's expectations about how variables under investigation are related are stated in the _____

    _____

11. The actual group of study participants selected from a larger group is known as the

    _____

12. The plan for transforming research information into a numerical format suitable for analysis is called the _____

13. The two broad classes of analysis are referred to as _____

    _____ and _____ analysis.

14. The final phase of a research project is known as the _____

    _____

15. The overall plan for collecting and analyzing scientific data is called the _____

    _____

16. The primary criterion by which a sample is assessed for adequacy is its _____

    _____

    of the population.

17. Typically, the most time-consuming phase of the study is the _____

    _____ phase.

18. The task of organizing the information collected in a study is known as _____

    _____

19. Research in which the investigator plays an active, interventive role is called

_____ research.

20. A variable that is irrelevant in an investigation and needs to be controlled is called

a(n) _____

_____

C. Study Questions

1. Define the following concepts. Compare your definition with the definition in Chapter 4 or in the glossary.

a. Variable: _____

_____

_____

b. Operational definition: _____

_____

_____

c. Heterogeneity: _____

_____

_____

d. Construct: _____

_____

_____

e. Dichotomous variable: _____

_____

_____

f. Relationship: _____

_____

_____

g. Cause-and-effect relationship: _____

_____

_____

h. Functional relationship: _____

_____

_____

i. Control: _____

_____

_____

2. Suggest operational definitions for the following concepts.

a. Stress: _____

_____

_____

b. Prematurity of infants: _____

_____

_____

c. Nursing effectiveness: _____

_____

_____

d. Knowledge of critical care nursing concepts: _____

_____

_____

e. Nurses' educational preparation: _____

_____

_____

f. Patient recovery: _____

_____

_____

g. Prolonged labor: _____

_____

_____

h. Nurses' professionalism: _____

_____

_____

i. Smoking behavior: _____

_____

_____

j. Nurses' job dissatisfaction: _____

_____

_____

k. Respiratory function: _____

_____

_____

l. Children's adjustment to hospitalization: _____

_____

_____

m. Patients' dependence levels: _____

_____

_____

3. In each of the following research problems, identify the independent and dependent variables.
   a. Does assertiveness training improve the effectiveness of psychiatric nurses?

   Independent: _____

   Dependent: _____
   b. Does the postural positioning of patients affect their respiratory function?

   Independent: _____

   Dependent: _____

c. Is the psychological well-being of patients affected by the amount of touch received from nursing staff?

Independent: _____

Dependent: _____

d. Is the incidence of decubiti reduced by more frequent turnings of patients?

Independent: _____

Dependent: _____

e. Is the educational preparation of nurses related to their subsequent turnover rate?

Independent: _____

Dependent: _____

f. Is tolerance for pain related to a patient's age and sex?

Independent: _____

Dependent: _____

g. Are the number of prenatal visits of pregnant women associated with labor and delivery outcomes?

Independent: _____

Dependent: _____

h. Are levels of stress among nurses higher in pediatric or adult intensive care units?

Independent: _____

Dependent: _____

i. Are student nurses' clinical grades related to their subsequent on-the-job performances?

Independent: _____

Dependent: _____

j. Is anxiety in surgical patients affected by structured preoperative teaching?

Independent: _____

Dependent: _____

k. Are nurses' promotions related to their level of participation in continuing education activities?

Independent: _____

Dependent: _____

l. Does hearing acuity of the elderly change as a function of the time of day?

Independent: _____

Dependent: _____

m. Is patient satisfaction with nursing care related to the congruity of nurses' and patients' cultural background?

Independent: _____

Dependent: _____

n. Is a woman's educational background related to breast self-examination practices?

Independent: _____

Dependent: _____

o. Does home birth affect the parents' satisfaction with the childbirth experience?

Independent: _____

Dependent: _____

4. Below is a list of variables. For each, think of a research problem for which the variable would be the independent variable, and a second for which it would be the dependent variable. For example, take the variable "birthweight of infants." We might ask, "Does the age of the mother affect the birthweight of her infant?" (dependent variable). Alternatively, we could define our research question as "Does the birthweight of infants (independent variable) affect their sensorimotor development at six months of age?" HINT: For the dependent variable problem, ask yourself, "What factors might affect, influence, or cause this variable?" For the independent variable, ask yourself, "What factors does *this* variable influence, cause, or affect?"

a. Body temperature

Independent: _____

Dependent: _____

b. Amount of sleep

Independent: _____

Dependent: _____

c. Attitudes toward nurse practitioners

Independent: _____

Dependent: _____

d. Participation in an HMO

Independent: _____

Dependent: _____
e. Amount of saliva secretion

Independent: _____

Dependent: _____
f. Nurses' absentee rate

Independent: _____

Dependent: _____

D. Application Exercises

Casertino (1991)* observed that different patients react differently to sensory overload in the hospital. She conducted a study to see whether the patients' home environments affect their reactions to hospital noises. Below are the investigator's operational definitions of the research variables.

Independent Variable: Type of home environment. Based on the patients' self-reports at intake, home environment was defined as the number of household members residing with the patient.

Dependent Variable: Reaction to hospital noise. Based upon responses to five questions (agree/disagree type) answered at discharge, patients were classified as "Dissatisfied with Noise Level" or "Not Dissatisfied with Noise Level."

Extraneous Variables

Age: calculated to the nearest year based on information on date of birth reported at intake

Sex: patient's gender as recorded on intake form

Social class: patient's occupation as recorded on intake form

1. Review and critique these specifications.† Suggest alternatives and compare the adequacy and completeness of your suggestions with the descriptions provided above. To aid you in this task, here are some guiding questions:

   a. Are the operational definitions sufficiently detailed? Do they tell the reader exactly how each variable is to be measured? Can you expand any of the definitions so that they are more precise?

---

*This example is fictitious.

†By "critique" we mean "assess," not criticize. That is, your critique should identify both positive and negative aspects.

    b. Are the operational definitions good definitions—that is, is there a better way to measure, say, home environment?

    c. Has the researcher identified reasonable extraneous variables—that is, are these extraneous variables likely to be related to both the dependent and independent variables?

    d. Are there extraneous variables that the researcher failed to identify but that should be controlled? Suggest two or three additional extraneous variables.

2. Below are several suggested research articles. Read one of these articles and respond to questions a to d from Question D.1 in critiquing this actual research study.

- Weaver, K.A. and Anderson, G.C. (1988). Relationship between integrated sucking pressures and first bottle-feeding scores in premature infants. *Journal of Obstetric, Gynecologic, and Neonatal Nursing, 17,* 113–120.

- White-Traut, R.C. and Nelson, M.N. (1988). Maternally administered tactile, auditory, visual, and vestibular stimulation. *Research in Nursing and Health, 11,* 31–39.

- Simpson, T. and Shaver, J. (1990). Cardiovascular responses to family visits in coronary care unit patients. *Heart and Lung, 19,* 344–351.

E. Special Projects

1. Suppose you were interested in studying the effect of a hysterectomy on women's sexuality and sexual identity. Briefly outline what you might do in the following tasks, as outlined in this chapter:

Step 4 Formulate hypotheses: _____

_____

_____

Step 5 Select a research design: _____

_____

_____

Step 6 Identify the population: _____

_____

_____

Step 7 Select measures/operationalize the variables: _____

_____

_____

Step 8 Select a sample: _____

_____

_____

2. Now suppose that, for the study you have described above, you needed to prepare a schedule for the completion of Steps 2 through 15. Assume you have 12 months to complete the study. Prepare a time schedule for the 14 tasks on the chart below:

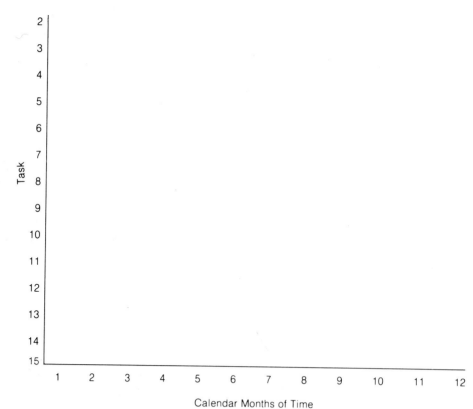

Calendar Months of Time

3. Another researcher is investigating the effect of auditory versus tactile stimulation on the crying behavior of premature infants. Ten babies are exposed to soft music for five minutes, four times a day. Ten other babies are exposed to extra touching and caressing for five minutes, four times a day. The dependent variable is the total number of minutes of crying among these infants for the five days of the treatment. Indicate a time schedule for this project, superimposed on the chart above, in a different color ink or pencil. Compare the differences between the two projects in time spent on various tasks. Justify the differences.

Part II

Preliminary Research Steps

5
Selecting and Defining a Nursing Research Problem

A. Matching Exercises

Match each problem statement in Set B with one of the phrases in Set A. Indicate the letter corresponding to the appropriate response next to each problem statement in Set B.

SET A
a. Statement in its current form represents a researchable, feasible problem.
b. Statement in its current form represents a researchable but unfeasible problem.
c. Statement in its current form represents an unresearchable problem.

SET B   **RESPONSE**

1. Are nurse practitioners better able to perform triage functions than physicians are?   _____

2. Do nurses need to carry professional liability insurance?   _____

3. The purpose of the study is to investigate the relationship between blood pressure readings and the incidence of cardiovascular accident in the elderly.   _____

4. Will the administration of two packs of cigarettes per day for 5 years result in lung cancer among a sample of nonsmokers?   _____

5. Should integrated-content curricula be adopted by baccalaureate nursing programs?   _____

6. Does method of suicide attempt vary according to the sex of the person? _____

7. Should all nursing students take a research methods course? _____

8. Does denial of prenatal care affect labor and delivery complications? _____

B. Completion Exercises

Write the words or phrases that correctly complete the sentences below.

1. The form of the problem statement can be either _____ _____ or _____ .

2. The four most common sources of ideas for research problems are _____ _____ , _____ , _____ , and _____ .

3. Unavailability of subjects would make a research project _____ _____ .

4. Moral or philosophical questions are inherently _____ _____ .

5. Adequacy of research facilities and time bear on the _____ _____ of the research project.

6. In order to be researchable, the variables in a research project need to be _____ .

C. Study Questions

1. Define the following terms. Compare your definition with the definition in Chapter 5 or in the glossary.

   a. Problem statement: _____

   _____

   _____

   b. Declarative problem statement: _____

   _____

   _____

   c. Interrogative problem statement: _____

_____

_____

   d. Unresearchable problem: _____

_____

_____

   e. Unfeasible problem: _____

_____

_____

2. Each of the problem statements below is either unresearchable or unfeasible as stated. Reword the statements, maintaining the general theme, such that a researchable and feasible problem is developed.

ORIGINAL	REWORDED
a. What is the best approach for dealing with family members of a dying patient?	_____
b. Should surrogate motherhood be forbidden by law?	_____
c. Should retirement for nurses be mandatory at age 65?	_____
d. Should abortion be available on demand?	_____
e. How can nurses be encouraged to do their own research?	_____
f. What is the best procedure for reducing stress among children prior to immunization?	_____
g. What incentives will motivate nursing faculty to publish professional articles?	_____
h. What role can humor play in improving the well-being of the institutionalized elderly?	_____

3. Below is a list of general topics that could be investigated. Develop at least one problem statement for each. Assess the adequacy of your statement in terms of the problem's researchability and feasibility. HINT: Think of these concepts as poten-

tial independent or dependent variables. Ask "What might cause or affect this variable?" and "What might be the consequences, or effects of this variable?" This should lead to some ideas for a problem statement. Also, review the question items in the section in the textbook called "Narrowing the Topic."

a. Patient comfort: _____

b. Psychiatric patients' readmission rates: _____

c. Anxiety in hospitalized children: _____

d. Oxytocin augmentation during labor: _____

e. Student attrition from nursing school: _____

f. Attitudes toward artificial insemination: _____

g. Incidence of venereal disease: _____

h. Requests for tubal ligation: _____

i. Elevated blood pressure: _____

_____

_____

j. Nurses' job satisfaction: _____

_____

_____

k. Patient cooperativeness in the recovery room: _____

_____

_____

l. Nutritional knowledge: _____

_____

_____

m. Mother–infant bonding: _____

_____

_____

n. Menstrual irregularities: _____

_____

_____

o. Accuracy of diagnosis: _____

_____

_____

4. Below is a list of researchable problem statements. Transform those stated in the interrogative form to the declarative form, and vice versa.

ORIGINAL VERSION	TRANSFORMED VERSION
a. Can a program of nursing counseling affect sexual readjustment among women following a hysterectomy?	_____
b. The purpose of the research is to study the relationship between nurses' unit assignments and their absentee rates.	_____

c. What are the sequelae of an inadequately maintained sterile environment for tracheal suctioning?

_____

d. What is the relationship between Type A/Type B personalities and speech patterns?

_____

e. The purpose of the study is to investigate the effect of a values clarification workshop on attitudes toward the mentally ill.

_____

f. The purpose of the research is to study patients' response to transfer from a coronary care unit to a general care unit.

_____

g. What effect does the presence of the father in the delivery room have upon the mother's satisfaction with the childbirth experience?

_____

h. The purpose of the study is to examine the effect of clients' physical proximity to community health centers on health care utilization.

_____

i. What is the long-term child-development effect of maternal heroin addiction during pregnancy?

_____

j. The purpose of the research is to study the effect of spermicides on the physiological development of the fetus.

_____

D. Application Exercises

Matysik (1990)* was interested in studying the effects of a mutual help group for widows and widowers. She designed a study in which 25 people who had lost a spouse 6 to 12 months earlier participated in biweekly mutual help group sessions. A comparison group of 25 nonparticipating widows and widowers was also included in the study. Matysik was interested in evaluating the effect of participation on several indices of socioemotional well-being. The purpose of her investigation was to answer the following questions:

*This example is fictitious.

- Does participation in a mutual help group improve the bereaved's morale?
- Does participation in a mutual help group reduce feelings of social isolation?
- Does participation in a mutual help group affect self-esteem?
- Does participation in a mutual help group lead to better acceptance of the spouse's death?

1. Review and critique these problem statements. Suggest alternatives and/or supplementary problem statements. To assist you, here are some guiding questions:

   a. How adequate are these problem statements in terms of researchability? Do they communicate the intent of the study? Can you alter the statements so that they are more precise or more amenable to research?

   b. Given the overall intent of the study, are the four specific problems a good, well-balanced representation? That is, are the four dependent variables good indicators of "socioemotional well-being"? Can you develop additional problem statements that would extend the overall goal of the project?

   c. What obstacles to the study's feasibility should the researcher consider?

2. Examine a recent issue of *Nursing Research*. Find an article that fails to provide a clearly articulated, concise problem statement. Write a problem statement for that article in either declarative or interrogative form.

E. Special Projects

1. Think of your clinical experience as a student or practicing nurse. Consider some aspect of your work that you particularly enjoy. Is there anything about that part of your work that puzzles, intrigues, or frustrates you? Can you conceive of any procedure, practice, or information that would improve the quality of your work in that area or improve the care you provide? Ask yourself a series of similar questions until a general problem area emerges. Narrow the problem area until you have a workable research problem statement. Assess the problem in terms of the criteria of significance, researchability, feasibility, and interest to you.

2. Read the article by Allen (1990) entitled "Physical and psychosocial outcomes after coronary artery bypass graft surgery," in *Heart and Lung, 19*, 49–54 (or read some other review article). Based on her summary of prior research, develop a problem statement for a study that would extend our knowledge about the outcomes associated with bypass surgery. Assess your problem statement in terms of the criteria of significance, researchability, feasibility, and personal interest.

6
Locating and Summarizing Existing Information on a Problem

A. Matching Exercises

Below, under Set B, are a number of fictitious references from the *International Nursing Index*. Identify the portion of the reference that is underlined and match it with a term in Set A. Indicate the letter corresponding to the appropriate response next to each entry in Set B.

SET A
a. Journal
b. Volume
c. Pages
d. Issue
e. Author
f. Title

SET B   **RESPONSE**

1. Convalescence following a hysterectomy. Mackey, K. <u>Nurs Res</u> 39(2): 157–162, Mar 90.

   _____

2. Nursing care program for bed-confined patients. <u>Gussman G.</u> Nurs Clin North Am 26(1): 83–96, Jan 91.

   _____

3. Nurse counseling following an abortion. Sala M. J Adv Nurs 9(6): 350–357, Nov 89. _____

4. Level of activation and respiratory function. Mosley M. Nurs Res 39(4): 196–202, July 90. _____

5. Holistic care in a community health center. Kamphaus M. Nurs Clin North Am 15(2): 101–115, Feb 87. _____

6. Treating bacteriuria in female patients with indwelling catheters. Porcelli P. Nurs Outlook 33(12):770–779, Dec 90. _____

7. Services for children with diabetes. Lewis O. Pediatrics 64(1): 15–20, Jan 85. _____

8. Screening for scoliosis in school-age children. Smith R. J. Sch Health 59(5): 315–319, May 89. _____

B. Completion Exercises

Write the words or phrases that correctly complete the sentences below.

1. The two types of information that have the least utility in a research review are

   _____ and _____ .

2. No hypothesis or theory can be definitively _____

   or _____ by the scientific method.

3. For students who are just beginning to engage in their own research, the most

   important function of the literature review will be as a source of _____

   _____ .

4. The most important type of information to be included in a written research

   review is _____

   _____ .

5. The oldest scholarly journal that has served as an outlet for nurses engaged in

   scientific research is _____

   _____ .

6. Quantity of references is less important in a good literature review than the __

   _____

   of the references.

7. The most relevant index for materials specific to nursing is the _____

   _____ .

8. When a computer search yields many references, the references are generally produced _____

   _____ .

9. The computer database most often used in literature searches by nurses is ____

   _____ .

10. The six sections typically found in research journal articles are:

    _____ , _____ , _____ ,

    _____ , _____ , and _____ .

11. The written literature review should paraphrase materials and use a minimum of

    _____ .

12. The literature review should make clear not only what is known about a problem

    but also any _____ in the research.

13. The review should conclude with a _____

    _____ .

14. The literature review should be written in a language of _____

    _____ ,

    in keeping with the limits of existing methods.

C. Study Questions

1. Define the following terms. Compare your definition with the definition in Chapter 6 of the textbook or in the glossary.

   a. Literature review: _____

   _____

   _____

   b. Primary source: _____

   _____

   _____

   c. Secondary source: _____

   _____

   _____

d. Computer search: _____

_____

_____

e. Index: _____

_____

_____

f. Abstract: _____

_____

_____

g. On-line search: _____

_____

_____

h. End-user system: _____

_____

_____

i. Journal article: _____

_____

_____

2. Below are fictitious excerpts from literature reviews. Each excerpt has a stylistic problem for a research review. Change each sentence to make it acceptable stylistically.

ORIGINAL	**REVISED**
a. Most elderly people do not eat a balanced diet.	_____
b. Patient characteristics have a significant impact on nursing workload.	_____
c. A child's conception of appropriate sick role behavior changes as the child grows older.	_____
d. Home birth poses many potential dangers.	_____

e. Multiple sclerosis results in considerable anxiety to the family of the patient.

_____

f. Studies have proven that most nurses prefer not to work the night shift.

_____

g. Life changes are the major cause of stress in adults.

_____

h. Stroke rehabilitation programs are most effective when they involve the patients' families.

_____

i. It has been proved that psychiatric outpatients have higher than normal rates of accidental deaths and suicides.

_____

j. Nursing faculty are increasingly involved in conducting their own research.

_____

k. Sickle cell counseling has emerged as an important service in community health centers.

_____

l. The traditional pelvic examination is sufficiently unpleasant to many women that they avoid having the examination.

_____

m. It is known that most tonsillectomies performed two decades ago were unnecessary.

_____

n. Few smokers seriously try to break the smoking habit.

_____

o. Severe cutaneous burns often result in hemorrhagic gastric erosions.

_____

3. Below are several problem statements. Indicate one or more terms or "keywords" that you would use to begin a literature search on this topic.

PROBLEM STATEMENT   **KEYWORDS**

a. How effective are nurse practitioners versus pediatricians with respect to telephone management of acute pediatric illness?

_____

b. Does contingency contracting improve patient compliance with a treatment regimen?

_____

c. Does induced abortion affect the outcome of subsequent pregnancies?

d. Is the amount of money a person spends on food related to the adequacy of nutrient intake?

e. Is rehabilitation following spinal cord injury affected by the age and social class of the patient?

f. Does the leadership style of head nurses affect the job tension and job performance of the nursing staff?

g. Is loss of appetite among cancer patients associated with reactions to chemotherapy?

h. What is the effect of alcohol skin preparation prior to insulin injection on the incidence of local and systemic infection?

i. Are bottle-fed babies introduced to solid foods sooner than breast-fed babies?

j. Do children raised on vegetarian diets have different growth patterns than do other children?

D. Application Exercises

Below is an excerpt from Gilboy's (1990)* literature review dealing with pelvic inflammatory disease.

There are no universally accepted criteria for defining pelvic inflammatory disease (PID) or for categorizing its severity. Furthermore, PID does not exhibit uniformity in its clinical features. Etiologically, cases of acute PID can be divided on the basis of those caused by *Neisseria gonorrhoeae,* those caused by nongonococcal bacteria, and those caused by a combination of both. Eschenbach and his colleagues (1980) have reported that approximately half of the women with PID whom they examined had gonococcal infections. Eschenbach (1982) has noted that "this difference in etiological agents may explain the clinical

*This example is fictitious.

differences between the gonococcal and nongonococcal PID. The latter may appear less acute and may not demonstrate many of the well-defined clinical features associated with gonorrhea" (p. 148). Both gonococcal and nongonococcal PID may result in subsequent obstruction of the Fallopian tubes, which is among the most common causes of infertility in women. Since fertilized eggs remain in the Fallopian tubes for approximately three days, they must provide nourishment for the developing zygote. Thus, even a tube which is not completely blocked, but which is severely damaged, can contribute to infertility.

Westrom (1979), in a study of women treated for PID, proved that PID has an impact on subsequent fertility. A sample of 415 women with laparoscopically confirmed PID were reviewed after 9.5 years and compared with 100 control subjects who had never been treated for PID. Among the 415 women who had had PID, 88 (21.2 percent) were involuntarily childless; of these 88, the failure to conceive was due to tubal obstruction in 72 cases (82 percent). A total of 263 of the 415 subjects (63.4 percent) had become pregnant. In the control group, only three women (three percent) were involuntarily childless.

Westrom's study also revealed a relationship between infertility and the number of PID infections. Tubal occlusion was diagnosed after one infection in 32 women (12.8 percent); after two infections in 22 cases (35.5 percent); and after three or more infections in 18 cases (75.0 percent). Of the 415 women with acute PID in Westrom's sample, 94 (22.7 percent) experienced more than one infection. Evidence from other studies confirms that a large percentage of women with PID have a history of previous PID, and that recurrent PID usually has a nongonococcal etiology (Jacobson and Westrom, 1974; Ringrose, 1970; Eschenbach, 1981).

The number of women affected by PID annually in the United States is unknown and difficult to estimate. According to Rose (1983), Eschenbach and colleagues used data from the National Disease and Therapeutic Index Study and the Hospital Record Study to estimate that over 500,000 cases of PID occurred annually in the United States in the early 1970s. The information from the Hospital Record Study indicated that a mean of over 160,000 patients with PID were hospitalized annually from 1970 through 1973.

1. Critique this literature review vis-à-vis the points made in Chapter 6 of the textbook. To assist you in this task, here are some guiding questions:

   a. Is the review well organized? Does the author skip from theme to theme in a disjointed way, or is there a logic to the order of presentation of materials?

   b. Is the content of the review appropriate? Does the author use secondary sources when a primary source was available? Are all of the references relevant, or does the inclusion of some material appear contrived? Do you have a sense that the author was thorough in uncovering all of the relevant materials? Do the references seem outdated? Is there an overdependence on opinion articles and/or anecdotes? Are prior studies merely summarized, or are their shortcomings discussed? Does the author indicate what is not known as well as what is?

   c. Does the style seem appropriate for a research review? Does the review seem biased or laden with subjective opinions? Is there too little paraphrasing and too much quoting? Does the author use appropriately tentative language in describing the results of earlier studies?

2. Read the literature review section in one of the articles listed below. Critique the review, applying questions a to c from Question D.1 above.

- Anderberg. G.J. (1988). Initial acquaintance and attachment behavior of siblings with the newborn. *Journal of Obstetric, Gynecologic, and Neonatal Nursing, 17,* 49–54.
- Aroian, K.J. (1990). A model of psychological adaptation to migration and resettlement. *Nursing Research, 39,* 5-9.
- Dimond, M., McCance, K., and King, K. (1987). Forced residential relocation: Its impact on the well-being of older adults. *Western Journal of Nursing Research, 9,* 445–464.
- Fortier, J.C. (1988). The relationship of vaginal and cesarean births to father-infant attachment. *Journal of Obstetric, Gynecologic, and Neonatal Nursing, 17,* 128–134.
- Wiley, K., Heath, L., Acklin, M., Earl, A., and Barnard, B. (1990). Care of HIV-infected patients. *Applied Nursing Research, 3,* 27–33.

E. Special Projects

1. Read the literature review section from a research article appearing in an issue of *Nursing Research* in the early 1980s (some possibilities are suggested below). Search the literature for more recent research on the topic of the article and update the review section. Don't forget to incorporate in your review the findings from the article itself! Here are some possible articles:

- Austin, J.K., McBride, A.B., and Davis, H.W. (1984). Parental attitude and adjustment to childhood epilepsy. *Nursing Research, 33,* 92–96.
- Choi-Lao, A. (1981). Trace anesthetic vapors in hospital operating-room environments. *Nursing Research, 30,* 156–161.
- Keane, A., Ducette, J., & Adler, D. (1985). Stress in ICU and non-ICU nurses. *Nursing Research, 34,* 231–236.

- Newport, M.A. (1984). Conserving thermal energy and social integrity in the newborn. *Western Journal of Nursing Research*, *6*, 175–188.
- Schraeder, B.D. and Cooper, B.M. (1983). Development and temperament in very low birth weight infants. *Nursing Research*, *32*, 331–335.

2. Select one of the problem statements from Question C.3, above. Conduct a literature search and identify five to ten relevant references. Compare your references with those of your classmates in terms of relevance, recency, and type of information provided.

3. Read one of the studies suggested in Question D.2. Write a two-page summary of the research report, translating the information into everyday (i.e., nonresearch) language.

7

Placing the Problem in a Theoretical Context

A. Matching Exercises

Match each statement from Set B with one of the phrases in Set A. Indicate the letter corresponding to your response next to each of the statements in Set B.

SET A
a. Theory
b. Conceptual framework
c. Model
d. Neither a, b, nor c
e. a, b, and c

SET B   **RESPONSE**

1. Makes minimal use of language   _____
2. Uses concepts as building blocks   _____
3. Is essential in the conduct of good research   _____
4. Can be used as a basis for generating hypotheses   _____
5. Can be proved through empirical testing   _____
6. Indicates a system of propositions that assert relationships among variables   _____
7. Is developed inductively through observations   _____

8. Consists of interrelated concepts organized in a rational scheme, but does not specify formal relationships among the concepts _____

9. Exists in nature and is awaiting scientific discovery _____

10. May help to stimulate new directions in research _____

B. Completion Exercises

Write the words or phrases that correctly complete the sentences below.

1. Theories are not found by scientists, they are _____

   _____ .

2. Deductions from theories are referred to as _____

   _____ .

3. Most of the conceptualizations of nursing practice would be called _____

   _____ .

4. Models attempt to represent reality with a minimal use of _____

   _____ .

5. $F = ma$ is an example of a(n) _____

   _____ .

6. In the statistical model $Y = \beta_1 X_1 + \beta_2 X_2 + e$, the βs are _____

   _____ .

7. The four central concepts of conceptual models in nursing are _____

   _____ , _____ , _____ , and _____ .

8. The basic intellectual process underlying theory development is _____

   _____ .

C. Study Questions

1. Define the following terms. Compare your definition with the definition in the glossary or in Chapter 7 of the textbook.

   a. Theory: _____

   _____

b. Macrotheory: _____

_____

_____

c. Middle-range theory: _____

_____

_____

d. Laws: _____

_____

_____

e. Conceptual framework: _____

_____

_____

f. Model: _____

_____

_____

g. Schematic model: _____

_____

_____

h. Statistical model: _____

_____

_____

i. Borrowed theory: _____

_____

_____

2. Read some recent issues of *Nursing Research* or another nursing research journal. Identify at least five different theories cited by nurse researchers in these research reports.

3. Using the statistical model presented in Chapter 7, suggest an alternative example for the Y (the dependent variable) and Xs the (independent variables). That is, hypothesize that some behavior or outcome of interest (Y) is due to the combined influence of four other factors (Xs).

4. Choose one of the eight conceptual frameworks of nursing that were described in this chapter. Develop a research hypothesis based on this framework.

5. Select one of the problem statements listed in Section C, question 4, from Chapter 5 of this Study Guide. Could your selected problem be developed within one of the eight nursing frameworks discussed in this chapter? Defend your answer.

D. Application Exercises

Webb (1991)* developed a study derived from Rotter's social learning theory. Social learning theory postulates that human behaviors are contingent upon the individual's expectancy that a particular behavior will be reinforced (rewarded). A key concept is locus of control, which is conceptualized as the degree to which a person perceives that rewards are a function of his or her own actions as opposed to external forces. Internal controllers are those who perceive themselves and their behavior as the major determinants of the reinforcement, while external controllers are those who tend to see little, if any, relationship between their own actions and subsequent reinforcement.

Webb hypothesized that individuals with an internal locus-of-control orientation would be more likely to engage in preventive health care activities than those with an external orientation. As a rationale for this hypothesis, she reasoned that "internal" people see themselves as capable of controlling health outcomes, while externally oriented people see forces outside of their control as the major determinants of health outcomes; the "externals" are, therefore, less likely to engage in preventive health care behaviors. To test her hypothesis, Webb operationalized "willingness to engage in preventive health care activities" as enrollment in a health maintenance organization among a group of employees who were offered a choice between a traditional medical benefits package and HMO membership. Five hundred employees hired by a large industrial firm

*This example is fictitious.

were administered a test that measured locus of control as part of the application process. Each new employee was offered a choice between the two medical programs. The 187 employees who chose HMO membership were found to have significantly higher (i.e., more internal) scores on the locus-of-control measure than the 313 employees who elected the traditional medical plan, thereby supporting Webb's hypothesis.

1. Review and critique the above study, particularly with respect to its theoretical basis. To assist you in your critique, here are some guiding questions:

   a. In what way, if any, did the use of a theory enhance the value of this study? Compare the meaningfulness of the study as described with what it would have been had the same hypothesis been tested in the absence of a theory.

   b. In what way, if any, did the outcome of the study affect the value of the theory? If the outcome had been different (e.g., no differences, or differences opposite to those predicted), what effect would that have had on the theory?

   c. Examine the study variables and hypothesis. Can you offer any suggestions for a different theoretical basis than the one used?

2. Read the introductory sections of one of the actual research studies cited below. Apply questions a–c from Question D.1 above to one of these studies.

   - Dodd, M. J. (1988). Patterns of self-care in patients with breast cancer. *Western Journal of Nursing Research, 10,* 7–24.

   - Gaydos, L.S. and Farnham, R. (1988). Human–animal relationships within the context of Rogers' principle of integrality. *Advances in Nursing Science, 10,* 72–80.

   - Henneman, E.A. (1989). Effect of nursing contact on the stress response of patients being weaned from mechanical ventilation. *Heart and Lung, 18,* 483–489.

   - Hughes, K.K. and Young, W.B. (1990). The relationship between task complexity and decision-making consistency. *Research in Nursing and Health, 13,* 189–197.

   - Lierman, L.M., Young, H.M., Kasprzyk, D., and Benoliel, J.Q. (1990). Predicting breast self-examination using the theory of reasoned action. *Nursing Research, 39,* 97–101.

   - McClowry, S.G. (1990). The relationship of temperament to pre- and posthospitalization behavioral responses of school-age children. *Nursing Research, 39,* 30–35.

E. Special Projects

1. One proposition of reinforcement theory is that *if* a behavior is rewarded (rein-forced), *then* the behavior will be repeated (learned). Based on this theory and on your observation of behaviors in health settings or schools of nursing, suggest three nursing research problem statements.

2. Select one of the problem statements in Table 5.2 of the textbook (or identify a problem statement of your own). Abstract a generalized issue (or several issues) from the statement. Search for an existing theory that might be applicable and appropriate.

3. Develop a researchable problem statement based on King's schematic model of the nursing process and interaction (Figure 7.1).

8
Formulating Hypotheses

A. Matching Exercises

Match each of the statements in Set B with one of the terms in Set A. Indicate the letter corresponding to the appropriate response next to each statement in Set B.

SET A
a. Research hypothesis—directional
b. Research hypothesis—nondirectional
c. Null hypothesis
d. Not a hypothesis as stated

SET B	**RESPONSE**
1. First-born infants have higher concentrations of estrogens and progesterone in umbilical cord blood than do later-born infants.	_____
2. There is no relationship between participation in prenatal classes and the health outcomes of infants.	_____
3. Nursing students are increasingly interested in obtaining advanced degrees.	_____
4. Nurse practitioners have more job mobility than do other registered nurses.	_____
5. A person's age is related to his or her difficulty in accessing health care.	_____
6. Glaucoma can be effectively screened by means of tonometry.	_____

7. Increased noise levels result in increased anxiety among hospitalized patients. _____

8. Media exposure of the health hazards of smoking is unrelated to the public's smoking habits. _____

9. Nurses' job satisfaction is correlated with levels of occupational stress. _____

10. The primary reason that nurses participate in continuing education programs is for professional advancement. _____

11. Baccalaureate, diploma, and associate degree nursing graduates differ with respect to technical and clinical skills acquired. _____

12. Nurses' experiences with abortion patients have no effect on the nurses' attitudes toward abortion. _____

13. Nurses' shift assignments are associated with their rates of absenteeism. _____

14. The presence of homonymous hemianopia in stroke patients negatively affects their length of stay in hospital. _____

15. Adjustment to hemodialysis does not vary by the patient's sex. _____

B. Completion Exercises

Write the words or phrases that correctly complete the sentences below.

1. Research hypotheses state a predicted _____

   _____ between variables.

2. Hypotheses normally should be formulated _____

   _____ data collection.

3. A hypothesis involves a prediction regarding at least _____

   _____ variables.

4. Another term for complex hypothesis is _____

   _____ .

5. Another term for a null hypothesis is _____

   _____ .

6. Hypotheses are generally tested by means of _____

_____ _____ .

7. Hypotheses predict the effect of the _____

variable on the _____ variable.

8. Theories often form the basis for _____

_____ hypotheses.

C. Study Questions

1. Define the following terms. Compare your definition with the definition in the glossary or in Chapter 8 of the textbook.

a. Hypothesis: _____

_____

_____

b. Inductive hypothesis: _____

_____

_____

c. Deductive hypothesis: _____

_____

_____

d. Simple hypothesis: _____

_____

_____

e. Complex hypothesis: _____

_____

_____

f. Nondirectional hypothesis: _____

_____

_____

g. Null hypothesis: _____

_____

_____

h. Directional hypothesis: _____

_____

_____

2. Below are five nondirectional hypotheses. Restate each one as a directional hypothesis.

NONDIRECTIONAL

a. Nurses' attitudes toward mental retardation vary according to their clinical specialty area.

b. Nurses and patients differ in terms of the relative importance they attach to having the patients' physical versus emotional needs met.

c. Nursing performance is rated differently by patients, family members of patients, and nursing supervisors.

d. ´ ne incidence of decubitus ulcers s related to the frequency of turning patients.

Baccalaureate and associate degree nurses differ in use of touch as a therapeutic device with patients.

DIRECTIONAL

a. _____

_____

b. _____

_____

c. _____

_____

d. _____

_____

e. _____

_____

Below are five simple hypotheses. Change each one to a complex hypothesis by adding either a dependent or independent variable.

SIMPLE HYPOTHESIS

a. First-time blood donors experience greater stress during the donation than donors who have given blood previously.

b. Nurses who initiate more conversation with patients are rated as more effective in their nursing care by patients than those who initiate less conversation.

COMPLEX HYPOTHESIS

a. _____

_____

b. _____

_____

c. Surgical patients who give high ratings to the informativeness of nursing communications experience less preoperative stress than do patients who give low ratings.

c. _____

_____

_____

d. Appendectomy patients whose peritoneums are drained with a Penrose drain will experience more peritoneal infection than patients who are not drained.

d. _____

_____

_____

e. Women who give birth by cesarean section are more likely to experience postpartum depression than women who give birth normally.

e. _____

_____

4. In study questions 2 and 3 above, ten research hypotheses were provided. Identify the independent and dependent variables in each.

INDEPENDENT VARIABLE(S)	DEPENDENT VARIABLES(S)
2a	
2b	
2c	
2d	
2e	
3a	
3b	
3c	
3d	
3e	

5. Below are five statements that are *not* research hypotheses as currently stated. Suggest modifications to these statements that would make them testable research hypotheses.

ORIGINAL STATEMENT

a. Relaxation therapy is effective in reducing hypertension.

b. The use of bilingual health care staff produces high utilization rates of health care facilities by ethnic minorities.

HYPOTHESIS

a. _____

_____

b. _____

_____

c. Nursing students are affected in their choice of clinical specialization by interactions with nursing faculty.

c. _____

_____

d. Sexually active teenagers have a high rate of using male methods of contraception.

d. _____

_____

e. In-use intravenous solutions become contaminated within 48 hours.

e. _____

_____

6. Review the three major purposes of a research hypothesis. In light of these purposes, explain why the null hypothesis is of less utility in the early phases of a scientific study than a research hypothesis.

D. Application Exercises

DelGiacco (1991)* was interested in studying the notes made by various members of the health care team on patients' hospital charts. The investigator was concerned with several aspects of the chart in terms of its communication potential to various hospital personnel. She began her project with some general questions, such as: Are the nurses' entries on the patient chart used by other staff? Who is most likely to read nurses' entries on the chart? Are there particular types of medical conditions that encourage staff utilization of nurses' entries? Do particular types of entries encourage utilization?

DelGiacco proceeded to reflect upon her own experiences and observations relative to these issues, and reviewed the literature to find whether other researchers had addressed these problems. Based on her review and reflections, DelGiacco developed the following hypotheses:

• Nursing notes on patients' charts are referred to infrequently by hospital personnel.

• Physicians refer to nursing notes on the patients' charts less frequently than do other personnel.

• The use of nursing notes by physicians is related to the location of the notes on the chart.

• Nurses perceive that nursing notes are referred to less frequently than they are in fact referred to.

• Nursing notes are more likely to be referred to by hospital personnel if the patient has been hospitalized for more than five days than if the patient has been hospitalized five days or fewer.

*This example is fictitious.

1. Review and critique these hypotheses. Suggest alternative wordings or supplementary hypotheses. To assist you, here are some guiding questions:

   a. Are all of the hypotheses testable as stated? What changes (if any) are needed to make all of the hypotheses testable?

   b. Are the hypotheses all consistent in format and style? That is, are they directional, nondirectional, or stated in the null form? Suggest changes, if appropriate, that would make them consistent.

   c. Are the above hypotheses reasonable (i.e., logical and consistent with your own experience and observations)? Are the hypotheses significant (i.e., do they have the potential to contribute to the nursing profession)?

   d. Based on the general problem that the researcher identified, can you generate additional hypotheses that could be tested? Can you suggest modifications to the hypotheses above to make them complex rather than simple (i.e., introduce additional independent or dependent variables)?

2. Below are several suggested research articles. Read the introductory sections of one or more of these articles and respond to questions a to d from Question D.1 in terms of these actual research studies:

   • Bliss-Holz, V.J. (1988). Primaiparas' prenatal concern for learning infant care. *Nursing Research*, 37, 20–21.

   • Cornwell, C.J. and Schmitt, M.H. (1990). Perceived health status, self-esteem and body image in women with rheumatoid arthritis or systemic lupus erythematosus. *Research in Nursing and Health*, 13, 99–107.

   • Deiriggi, P.M. (1990). Effects of waterbed flotation on indicators of energy expenditure in preterm infants. *Nursing Research*, 39, 140–146.

   • Lanza, M.L. (1988). Reactions of nurses to a patient assault vignette. *Western Journal of Nursing Research*, 10, 45–54.

E. Special Projects

1. Below are two sets of variables. Select a variable from each set to generate directional hypotheses. In other words, use one variable in Set A as the independent variable and one variable in Set B as the dependent variable (or vice versa), and make a prediction about the relationship between the two.* Generate five hypotheses in this fashion.

SET A	SET B
body temperature	patient satisfaction with nursing care
nursing students' drop-out rate	nurses' educational preparation

*As one example: Pregnant women who smoke will give birth to babies with lower Apgar scores than women who do not smoke.

attitudes toward death

frequency of medications

delivery by nurse midwife versus physician

participation in continuing education courses

years of nursing experience

amount of interaction between nurses and patients' families

preoperative anxiety levels

patients' amount of privacy during hospitalization

amount of smoking

recidivism in a psychiatric hospital

infant Apgar score

attitudes toward nursing research

effectiveness of nursing care

nursing specialty area

patients' compliance with nursing instructions

nurses' part-time versus full-time work schedules

nurses' ages

nurses' empathy

hospital staff morale

patients' pulse rates

2. Prepare your own lists of variables from which hypotheses could be generated. Develop five more hypotheses based on your lists.

3. Assess the hypotheses generated in either Exercise E.1 or E.2 in terms of significance, testability, and interest to you.

Part III

Designs for Nursing Research

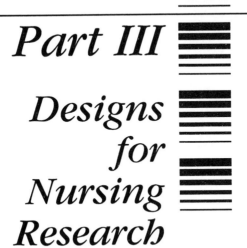

9
Experiments and Quasi-Experiments

A. Matching Exercises

Match each type of design from Set A with one (or more) of the representations from Set B. Indicate the letter corresponding to your response next to each item in Set A.

SET A   **RESPONSE**

1. True experimental design   _____

2. Time-series design   _____

3. Nonequivalent control group pretest/posttest design   _____

4. Pre-experimental design   _____

SET B

a. $\underline{\quad X \qquad O \quad}$
$\qquad\qquad\quad O$

b. $O_1 O_2 O_3 O_4 \quad X \quad O_5 O_6 O_7 O_8$

c. $\underline{R \quad X \qquad O}$
$\quad R \qquad\qquad O$

d. $\underline{O_1 \quad X \qquad O_2}$
$\quad O_1 \qquad\qquad O_2$

e. $O_1 \quad X \qquad O_2$

f. $R \quad O_1 \quad X_1 \quad O_2$
$\underline{R \quad O_1 \quad X_2 \quad O_2}$
$R \quad O_1 \qquad\qquad O_2$

g. Time 1
$\underline{O_1 O_2 \qquad\qquad\qquad}$
$\qquad\qquad$ Time 2
$\qquad\quad O_1 \quad X \quad O_2$

h. $O_1 \quad O_2 \quad O_3 \quad O_4 \quad X \quad O_5 \quad O_6 \quad O_7 \quad O_8$
$O_1 \quad O_2 \quad O_3 \quad O_4 \qquad\quad O_5 \quad O_6 \quad O_7 \quad O_8$

B. Completion Exercises

Write the words or phrases that correctly complete the sentences below.

1. In an experiment, the researcher manipulates the _____ variable.
2. The manipulation that the researcher introduces is referred to as the experimental _____

   _____.
3. Randomization is performed so that groups will be formed without _____

   _____.
4. When more than one independent variable is being simultaneously manipulated

   by the researcher, the design is referred to as a(n) _____

   _____.
5. The most typical method of randomization is through the use of a(n) _____

   _____.
6. Each factor in an experimental design must have two or more _____

   _____.
7. A primary objective of a true experiment is to enable the researcher to infer

   _____.
8. When a true experimental design is not used, the control group is usually referred

   to as the _____ group.
9. A research design that lacks the controls of a quasi-experiment is referred to as

   a(n) _____ design.
10. A quasi-experimental design that involves repeated observations over time is

    referred to as the _____

    _____.
11. Another term for randomization is _____ .
12. When data are gathered prior to the institution of some treatment, the initial data

    gathering is referred to as the _____ .
13. When neither the subjects nor the persons collecting data know in which group a

    subject is participating, the procedures are called _____ .
14. The difficulty with a nonequivalent control group design is that the experimental

    and comparison groups cannot be assumed to be _____

    _____ prior to the intervention.

C. *Study Questions*

1. Define the following terms. Compare your definition with the definition in the glossary or in Chapter 9 of the textbook.

   a. Experiment: _____

   _____

   _____

   b. Manipulation: _____

   _____

   _____

   c. Randomization: _____

   _____

   _____

   d. Control group: _____

   _____

   _____

   e. Clinical trial: _____

   _____

   _____

   f. Solomon four-group design: _____

   _____

   _____

   g. Interaction effects: _____

   _____

   _____

   h. Hawthorne effect: _____

   _____

   _____

   i. Quasi-experiment: _____

   _____

   _____

j. Rival hypothesis: _____

_____

_____

2. Below are 20 subjects who have volunteered for a study of the effects of noise on pulse rate. Ten must be assigned to the low-volume group and ten to a high-volume group. Use the table of random numbers in Table 9-1 of the text to randomly assign subjects to groups and groups to treatments.

J. Foster	C. Prodromos	S. Dunne	J. Sinar
M. Higley	J. Kurz	W. Niro	R. Phelps
J. Enright	C. Pananelli	B. Hakan	E. Stautner
K. Clements	G. Nudo	B. Schwing	J. Trice
J. Valek	J. Lamphier	J. Traetta	J. McGregor

3. Assume all of the subjects in the first two columns above are in their 20s and all the subjects in the last two columns are in their 30s. How good a job did your randomization do in terms of equalizing the experimental and control groups according to age? Add ten more names to each age group and assign these additional 20 subjects. Now compare the low-volume and high-volume groups in terms of the age distribution. Did doubling the sample size improve the distribution of the subjects' ages within the two volume-level groups?

4. Read one of the articles listed under "Substantive References" in Chapter 9 of the textbook. Using the notation presented in Figures 9-4 to 9-13, diagram the research design of the study.

D. Application Exercises

Kross (1990)* wanted to test the effectiveness of a new relaxation/biofeedback intervention on menopause symptoms. She invited women who presented themselves in an outpatient clinic with complaints of severe hot flashes to participate in the study of the experimental treatment. These 30 women were asked to record, every day for one week prior to their treatment, the frequency and duration of their hot flashes. During the intervention, which involved six one-hour sessions over a three-week period, the women again recorded their symptoms. Then, four weeks after the treatment, the women were asked to record their hot flashes over a five-day period. At the end of the study, Kross found that both the frequency and average duration of the hot flashes had been

*This example is fictitious.

significantly reduced in this sample of women. She concluded that her new treatment was an effective alternative to estrogen replacement therapy in treating menopausal hot flashes.

1. Review and critique this study. Suggest alternative designs for testing the effectiveness of the treatment. To assist you in your critique, here are some guiding questions:

    a. Is the design described above experimental, quasi-experimental, or pre-experimental? Diagram the design using the notation shown in Figures 9-4 to 9-13 of the text.

    b. The investigator concluded that the outcome (i.e., the reduction in the frequency and duration of the women's hot flashes) was attributable to the experimental treatment. Can you offer one or more alternative explanations to account for the outcome? Discuss the inference of causality in the context of this research design.

    c. Consider your responses to part b above. If you have identified any weaknesses in the design of this research, suggest a modified design that would improve the study. In what way does your new design eliminate the problems of the original design?

2. Below are several suggested research articles. Read one or more of these articles and respond to questions a to d from Question D.1 in terms of these actual research studies.

    • Fegley, B.J. (1988). Preparing children for radiologic procedures: Contingent versus noncontingent instruction. *Research in Nursing and Health, 11*, 3–9.
    • Keefe, M.R. (1988). The impact of infant rooming-in on maternal sleep at night. *Journal of Obstetric, Gynecologic, and Neonatal Nursing, 17*, 122–126.
    • Naylor, M.D. (1990). Comprehensive discharge planning for hospitalized elderly: A pilot study. *Nursing Research, 39*, 156–161.
    • Stevenson, J.S. and Topp, R. (1990). Effects of moderate and low intensity long-term exercise by older adults. *Research in Nursing and Health, 13*, 209–218.
    • Weinbacher, F.M., Littlejohn, C.E., and Conley, P.F. (1990). Growth of bacteria in prefilled syringes stored in home refrigerators. *Applied Nursing Research, 3*, 63–67.

E. Special Projects

1. Suppose that you were interested in testing the hypothesis that a regular regimen of exercise reduces blood pressure, improves cardiovascular efficiency, and increases coronary circulation. Design a quasi-experiment to test the hypothesis.

Evaluate this design vis-à-vis the ability to make causal inferences. Design a true experiment to test the same hypothesis and compare the kinds of conclusions that can be drawn with this design with those from the quasi-experiment.

2. Generate a hypothesis of your own in which the aim is to establish a cause-and-effect relationship. Design both a quasi-experiment and a true experiment and compare how the designs address possible alternative explanations of the results.

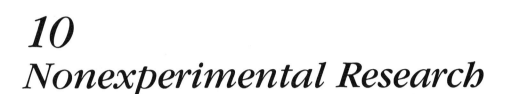

10
Nonexperimental Research

A. *Matching Exercises*

Match each problem statement from Set B with one (or more) of the phrases from Set A that indicates a potential reason for using a nonexperimental approach. Indicate the letter(s) corresponding to your response next to each statement in Set B.

SET A
a. Independent variable not manipulable
b. Ethical constraints on manipulation
c. Practical constraints on manipulation
d. No constraints on manipulation

SET B   **RESPONSE**

1. Does the use of certain tampons cause toxic shock syndrome?   _____

2. Does heroin addiction among mothers affect Apgar scores of
   infants?   _____

3. Is the age of a hemodialysis patient related to the incidence of
   the disequilibrium syndrome?   _____

4. What body positions aid respiratory function?   _____

5. Does the ingestion of saccharin cause cancer in humans?   _____

6. Is a nurse's attitude toward the elderly related to his or her
   choice of a clinical specialty?   _____

7. Does the use of touch by nursing staff affect patient morale?   _____

8. Does a nurse's gender affect his or her salary and rate of promotion? _____

9. Does extreme athletic exertion in young women cause amenorrhea? _____

10. Does assertiveness training affect a psychiatric nurse's job performance? _____

B. Completion Exercises

Write the words or phrases that correctly complete the sentences below.

1. In ex post facto research, the investigator forfeits control over the _____ _____ variable.

2. In ex post facto research, it is difficult, if not impossible, to establish _____ _____ relationships.

3. Some forms of ex post facto research are referred to as _____ _____ research.

4. Correlation does not prove _____ _____ .

5. When no variable is manipulated in a study, the research is called _____ _____ .

6. A prospective design is more rigorous in elucidating casual relations than a _____ design.

7. In ex post facto research, when two groups are compared in terms of some outcome, the groups are *not* formed by means of _____ _____ .

8. One major advantage of correlational research is its ability to collect large amounts of _____ _____ .

9. The fallacy of "post hoc ergo propter" lies in an assumption that one thing caused another simply because the presumed cause _____ the presumed effect.

10. Because ex post facto studies tend to be conducted in natural settings, one advantage of them is that they are strong in _____

_____ .

C. *Study Questions*

1. Define the following terms. Compare your definition with the definition in Chapter 10 of the textbook or in the glossary.

   a. Ex post facto research: _____

   _____

   _____

   b. Retrospective study: _____

   _____

   _____

   c. Prospective study: _____

   _____

   _____

   d. Path analysis: _____

   _____

   _____

   e. Mediating variable: _____

   _____

   _____

   f. Prediction study: _____

   _____

   _____

   g. Nonexperimental research: _____

   _____

   _____

  h. Univariate descriptive study: _____

  _____

  _____

  i. Self-selection: _____

  _____

  _____

  j. Post hoc ergo propter: _____

  _____

  _____

2. A nurse researcher found a relationship between teenagers' level of knowledge about birth control and their level of sexual activity. That is, teenagers with higher levels of sexual activity knew more about birth control than teenagers with less sexual activity. Suggest at least three interpretations for this finding.

  a. _____

  _____

  _____

  b. _____

  _____

  _____

  c. _____

  _____

  _____

3. Does Exercise 2 above describe a research problem that is *inherently* nonexperimental? Why or why not?

4. Which of the following variables *inherently* cannot be manipulated by a researcher?*

	CAN BE MANIPULATED	CANNOT BE MANIPULATED
a. Age at onset of obesity	_____	_____
b. Amount of auditory stimulation	_____	_____

*Remember that *manipulation* does not refer to whether or not the variable can be *affected* by a researcher; it refers to the researcher's ability to randomly assign individuals to different levels of the variable or to different groups.

    c. Number of cigarettes smoked   _____   _____

    d. Infant's birthweight   _____   _____

    e. Blood type   _____   _____

    f. Preoperative anxiety   _____   _____

    g. Type of nursing curriculum   _____   _____

    h. Attitudes toward nurses' extended role   _____   _____

    i. Nurses' shift assignments   _____   _____

    j. Type of birth control method used   _____   _____

    k. Mother–infant bonding   _____   _____

    l. Use of A-V shunt versus A-V fistula   _____   _____

    m. Fluid intake   _____   _____

    n. Morale of dying patients' family members   _____   _____

    o. Nurses' fringe benefits   _____   _____

5. A researcher has found that supervisors' ratings of nurses' job performance are related to the nurses' self-reported job satisfaction. That is, nurses who receive higher job evaluations are more satisfied than nurses with lower ratings. Suggest at least three interpretations for this result.

    a. _____

    _____

    _____

    b. _____

    _____

    _____

    c. _____

    _____

    _____

6. Does Exercise 5 above describe a research problem that is *inherently* nonexperimental? Why or why not?

7. Refer to the ten hypotheses in Exercises C.2 and C.3 of Chapter 8. Indicate below whether these hypotheses could be tested using an experimental/quasi-experimental approach, a nonexperimental approach, or both.

	EXPERIMENTAL/ QUASI-EXPERIMENTAL	NONEXPERIMENTAL	BOTH
2a	_____	_____	_____
2b	_____	_____	_____
2c	_____	_____	_____
2d	_____	_____	_____
2e	_____	_____	_____
3a	_____	_____	_____
3b	_____	_____	_____
3c	_____	_____	_____
3d	_____	_____	_____
3e	_____	_____	_____

8. Can most problems that are researched using an experimental approach be researched using a nonexperimental approach? How about vice versa? Why or why not?

D. Application Exercises

Buffington (1991)* hypothesized that the absence of socioemotional supports among the elderly results in a high level of chronic health problems and low morale. She tested this hypothesis by interviewing a sample of 250 residents of one community who were aged 65 and older. The respondents were randomly selected from a list of town residents. Buffington used several measures regarding the availability of social/emotional supports: (1) whether the respondent lived with any kin; (2) whether the respondent had any living children who resided within 30 minutes away; (3) the total number of interactions the respondent had had in the previous week with kin not residing in his or her household; and (4) the number of close friends in whom the respondent felt he or she could confide. Based on responses to the various questions on social support, respondents were classified in one of three groups: low social support, moderate social support, and high social support.

*This example is fictitious.

In a six-month follow-up interview, Buffington collected information from 214 respondents about the frequency and intensity of the respondents' illnesses in the preceding six-months, their hospitalization record, their overall satisfaction with life, and their attitudes toward their own aging. An analysis of the data revealed that the low-support group had significantly more health problems, lower life satisfaction ratings, and lower acceptance of their aging than the other two groups. Buffington concluded that the availability of social supports resulted in better physical and mental adjustment to old age.

1. Review and critique this study. Suggest alternative designs for testing the researcher's hypothesis. To assist you in your critique, here are some guiding questions:

   a. Is this research nonexperimental? If so, is it *inherently* nonexperimental? Why or why not? If so, what *type* of nonexperimental research is it?

   b. Examine the criteria for causality presented in Chapter 9 of the text. Does this study meet all of the criteria for establishing causality?

   c. The researcher concluded that her independent variable (amount of social support) "caused" certain outcomes (mental and physical health status in the elderly). Can you offer two or more alternative explanations to account for the outcome?

   d. Consider your responses to parts b and c above. If you have identified any weaknesses in the design of this research, suggest modifications that would improve the study design.

2. Below are several suggested research articles. Read the introductory and methods sections of one or more of these articles and respond to questions a to d from Question D.1 in terms of these actual research studies.

   • Keltner, B., Keltner, N.L. and Farren, E. (1990). Family routines and conduct disorders in adolescent girls. *Western Journal of Nursing Research*, *12*, 161–174.

   • Murphy, S.A. (1988). Mental distress and recovery in a high-risk bereavement sample three years after untimely death. *Nursing Research*, *37*, 30–35.

   • Schraeder, B.D., Heverty, M.A., and Rappaport, J. (1990). Temperament, behavior problems, and learning skills in very low birth weight preschoolers. *Research in Nursing and Health*, *13*, 27–34.

   • Sexton, D.L. and Munro, B.H. (1988). Living with a chronic illness. *Western Journal of Nursing Research*, *10*, 26–38.

E. Special Projects

1. Refer to Exercise E.1 in Chapter 9. Describe how you might design an ex post facto study to test the same hypothesis.

2. Generate a problem statement for each of the types of nonexperimental research (e.g., retrospective, prospective, etc.) described in Chapter 10 of the text.

3. Suppose that you were interested in testing the hypothesis that the use of IUDs could cause infertility. Describe how such a hypothesis could be tested using a retrospective design. Now describe a prospective design for the same study. Compare the strengths and weaknesses of the two approaches. Could an experimental or quasi-experimental design be used? Why or why not?

11
Additional Types of Research

A. *Matching Exercises*

Match each problem statement from Set B with one (or more) of the types of research that could be undertaken to address the problem listed in Set A. Indicate the letter(s) corresponding to your response next to each of the statements in Set B.

SET A
a. Survey research
b. Field research
c. Evaluation research
d. Needs assessment
e. Historical research
f. Case study
g. Methodological research

SET B	RESPONSE
1. What type of social and health services are needed by the rural elderly?	_____
2. Does the assurance of anonymity to respondents increase self-reports of socially undesirable behavior such as child or spouse abuse?	_____
3. Do parents approve of sex education in the schools?	_____

4. Can a new curriculum improve students' scores on the licen-
sure examination at the Eastern University's School of
Nursing?   _____

5. What is the effect of social change regarding men's and wom-
en's roles on the image of male nurses?   _____

6. Are patients' ratings of nurses' job performance less accurate
than supervisors' ratings?   _____

7. Is a radio-based media campaign more effective than a
print-based media campaign in recruiting blood donors?   _____

8. How does a community react to the stress of a natural disaster
such as a hurricane?   _____

9. How do nursing faculty feel about the inclusion of nursing
research courses in the undergraduate curriculum?   _____

10. Does the block rotation method of scheduling result in a
lower absentee rate among nursing staff than a random rotation method?   _____

B. Completion Exercises

Write the words or phrases that correctly complete the sentences below.

1. Surveys rarely involve questioning an entire _____
_____ , but rely instead on samples.

2. Interviews via the _____
_____ are less expensive than in-person interviews.

3. When a survey instrument is self-administered, it is referred to as a(n) _____
_____ .

4. Studies of individuals in naturalistic social settings are referred to as _____
_____ .

5. In evaluation research, behavioral objectives should focus on the behavior of the
_____
of a program, not the agents.

6. Program evaluations that do not focus exclusively on intended outcomes but that
consider broader, unintended ones as well are often referred to as _____
_____ .

7. Evaluations that focus on the net effects of an intervention are referred to as

   _____ .

8. A _____

   is a form of evaluation undertaken to determine the financial effects of a program.

9. The method of collecting needs assessment data by questioning knowledgeable

   individuals is known as the _____

   _____ .

10. In historical research, first-hand accounts of events or experiences are referred to

    as _____

    _____ .

11. Historical researchers who question the authenticity of a document or artifact are

    invoking _____

    _____ criticism.

12. Secondary analysis involves the use of previously collected _____

    _____ .

13. When a researcher analyzes data as a secondary analysis and either aggregates

    or disaggregates the data differently, we say that there has been a change in the

    _____ .

14. In meta-analyses, the index that is calculated for each study to summarize the

    magnitude of group differences is the _____

    _____ .

15. Methodological research is so named because it is research conducted for the

    purpose of developing or refining research _____

    _____ .

C. Study Questions

1. Define the following terms. Compare your definition with the definition in Chapter 11 of the textbook or in the glossary.

   a. Survey research: _____

   _____

   _____

   b. Personal interview: _____

   c. Census:

   d. Ethnonursing research:

   e. Evaluation research: _____

   f. Summative evaluation: _____

   g. Process evaluation:

   h. Policy research:

   i. Needs assessment: _____

   j. Indicators approach:

   k. Historical research: _____

l. Case study: _____

_____

_____

m. Secondary analysis: _____

_____

_____

n. Meta-analysis: _____

_____

_____

o. Methodological research: _____

_____

_____

2. Suppose that you were interested in studying the problems below by means of a survey. For each, indicate whether you would recommend using a personal interview, a telephone interview, or a questionnaire to collect the data. Justify your response.

   a. How well informed are nursing students about venereal disease? _____

   b. What are the coping strategies and behaviors of newly widowed individuals? _____

   c. What is the attitude of the general population toward HMOs? _____

   d. What are the emotional sequelae of having an organ transplant? _____

   e. Do nursing faculty in different clinical specialties differ in their scholarly productivity? _____

   f. Are nurses' attitudes toward unionization related to their incomes? _____

   g. Are the rural elderly more socially isolated than the urban elderly? _____

   h. Are people's attitudes toward "test tube babies" related to their religious affiliation? _____

    i. Is the "socialization process" for new nursing graduates in their first job smoother in large or small hospitals? _____

    j. What type of nursing communications do presurgical patients find most helpful? _____

3. Listed below are several "programs" or policies that could be evaluated. Think of one or more objectives that such a program might have that would be amenable to evaluation and state them as *behavioral* objectives. Remember that it is the intended behavior of *recipients* that must be specified.

    a. A continuing education workshop on new techniques in monitoring intracranial pressure.

    b. Nurses' instructions to dialysis patients regarding the hygienic care of their shunt.

    c. A crisis intervention program for rape victims.

    d. A new fringe benefit package for nursing staff.

    e. An instructional unit that teaches techniques in respiratory assessment to nursing students.

4. Below are several research problems. Indicate for each whether you think the problem should be studied using a survey approach or a field study approach. Justify your response.

    a. By what process do new nursing home residents learn to adapt to their environments?

    b. What aspects of their jobs are related to job satisfaction among school nurses?

    c. What is the relationship between a teenager's health-risk appraisal and various forms of risk-taking behavior (e.g., smoking, sexual activity without contraception, using drugs, etc.)?

    d. What aspects of the lifestyles of urban disadvantaged women place them at especially high risk of pregnancy and childbirth complications?

    e. How are the dynamics of nurse–patient interaction affected by the presence of a physician?

5. Are the problems that survey researchers address usually amenable to experimentation? Why or why not? How about the studies undertaken by field researchers?

6. A nurse researcher is developing a study to evaluate the effectiveness of a program that uses nurse practitioners to manage common respiratory infections. Suggest a design for an impact analysis.

7. Consider a client group of interest to you. Suggest an approach for conducting a needs assessment for this group.

8. Suppose you were interested in conducting a case study on a person with insomnia. Describe what your approach would be. What types of data would you collect? What might some of the ethical considerations of such a study be?

9. Read the methodological study by Miller and Powers (1988) in *Nursing Research*, volume 37, pages 6–10. Design at least one substantive study that would use their measure of hope as the dependent variable.

D. Application Exercises

Marter (1991)* studied the contraceptive practices of university students at three large midwestern universities. In addition to obtaining descriptive information, he wanted to test the hypothesis that students who report favorable experiences with health-care personnel relating to contraceptives are more likely than those with unfavorable experiences to practice birth control effectively. A random sample of 500 students from each university were sent a mailed questionnaire. A total of 715 usable questionnaires was returned. The questionnaire included questions on sexual experience, contraceptive use history, perceived ease of access to birth control, feelings about seeking out contraceptive information, knowledge of on-campus contraceptive services, and experiences with health-care personnel related to contraceptives. The questionnaire also asked about the student's age, ethnicity, year in college, major, father's occupation, marital status, religion, and grade point average. Marter's data revealed that while the majority of students were sexually experienced, fewer than half had used any birth control during their last intercourse. Approximately 60 percent of the sexually active students had had a contact with health-care personnel relating to

*This example is fictitious.

contraceptives, and of these, 70 percent described their experience in positive terms. In comparing those who had had favorable and unfavorable experiences, Marter found that a significantly higher percentage of those with a favorable experience (68 percent versus 42 percent) had used some form of contraceptive at last intercourse. He concluded that a favorable experience with health-care personnel leads to better contraceptive utilization. He speculated that those with more positive experiences were better informed about and more accepting of contraception than those with negative experiences and hence practiced birth control more conscientiously.

1. Review and critique this study. Suggest alternative methods for conducting this research. To assist you in your critique, here are some guiding questions:
   a. Is this research nonexperimental? If so, is it *inherently* nonexperimental? Why or why not?
   b. What type of research study is this, in terms of the types discussed in this chapter? Could the same research problem be studied using an alternative approach (i.e., one of the other types of research discussed in the chapter)?
   c. Examine the criteria for causality presented in Chapter 9 of the text. Does this study meet all of the criteria for establishing causality?
   d. The researcher concluded that the independent variable (quality of the students' experience with health-care personnel) "caused" a certain outcome (contraceptive utilization). Can you offer two or more alternative explanations to account for the outcome?
   e. Consider your responses to parts b and c, above. If you have identified any weaknesses in the design of this research, suggest modifications that would improve the study design.
   f. Consider the investigator's method of data collection. What problems, if any, does this data collection method pose for this research? Would you recommend an alternative method? Why or why not?
   g. Prepare two or three hypotheses that you could test in a secondary analysis of this researcher's data.

2. Below are several suggested research articles. Skim one or more of these articles and respond to questions a through g from Question D.1 in terms of this actual research study.

   • Church, O. M. (1987). From custody to community in psychiatric nursing. *Nursing Research, 36*, 48–55.
   • Katzman, E. M. and Roberts, J. I. (1988). Nurse–physician conflicts as barriers to the enactment of nursing roles. *Western Journal of Nursing Research, 10*, 576–590.
   • Reis, J. (1990). Medicaid maternal and child health care: Prepaid vs. private fee-for-service. *Research in Nursing and Health, 13*, 163–171.

- Slager-Earnest, S. E., Hoffman, S. J., and Beckman, C.J.A. (1987). Effects of a specialized prenatal adolescent program on maternal and infant outcomes. *Journal of Obstetric, Gynecologic, and Neonatal Nursing, 16,* 422–429.
- White, M. A., Williams, P. D., Alexander, D. J., Powell-Cope, G. M., and Conlon, M. (1990). Sleep onset latency and distress in hospitalized children. *Nursing Research, 39,* 134–139.
- Young, C., McMahon, J. E., Bowman, V., and Thompson, D. (1989). Maternal reasons for delayed prenatal care. *Nursing Research, 38,* 242–243.

E. Special Projects

1. Generate one problem statement for each of the following types of research that were described in this chapter.

   a. Survey research: _____

   _____

   _____

   b. Field research: _____

   _____

   _____

   c. Evaluation research: _____

   _____

   _____

   d. Needs assessment: _____

   _____

   _____

   e. Case study: _____

   _____

   _____

   f. Historical research: _____

   _____

   _____

2. Identify a problem amenable to survey research that you would be interested in studying. Outline the *kinds* of information you would want to collect in the survey (e.g., What types of background information?). Would you use personal interviews, telephone interviews, or questionnaires to collect your data? Why? Could the same problem be studied using field research methods? Why or why not?

3. Suppose that you were interested in studying a community's need for a food supplement program for low-income pregnant women. How could you use the key informant approach, the survey approach, and the indicator approach to research this problem? Which approach do you think would yield the most meaningful data? Why?

4. Read Tulman and Fawcett's (1990) article entitled "Maternal employment following childbirth," which appeared in volume 13 of *Research in Nursing and Health* (pp. 181–188). Generate several hypotheses that could be tested by means of a secondary analysis of their data set.

12
Principles of Research Design

A. Matching Exercises

Match each "threat" from Set B with a phrase from Set A that indicates the nature of the "threat." Indicate the letter corresponding to your response next to each statement in Set B.

SET A
a. Internal validity
b. External validity
c. Neither internal nor external validity

SET B	**RESPONSE**
1. Selection effects	_____
2. Maturation effects	_____
3. Manipulation	_____
4. Novelty effects	_____
5. Replication	_____
6. Testing	_____
7. Hawthorne effect	_____
8. Experimenter effects	_____
9. Blocking effects	_____
10. Mortality	_____

B. Completion Exercises

Write the words or phrases that correctly complete the sentences below.

1. Research design is concerned with maximizing the researcher's _____ _____ .

2. The environment should be controlled by the researcher insofar as possible by maximizing _____ _____ in the research conditions.

3. The specifications of an experimental treatment are often referred to as the _____ .

4. Randomization serves a general control function in research design by eliminating _____ .

5. Using the principle of homogeneity to control extraneous variables limits the _____ of the findings.

6. When an extraneous variable is dealt with in a randomized block design, the variable is then referred to as a(n) _____ variable.

7. When a repeated measures design is used, the procedure of _____ _____ should usually be employed to counteract any ordering effects.

8. The research procedure that controls all possible extraneous variables when two or more groups are involved is known as _____ .

9. Control over extraneous variables is required for the _____ _____ validity of the study.

10. The differential loss of subjects from comparison groups is the threat known as _____ .

11. Changes that occur as the result of time passing rather than as a result of the treatment represent the threat of _____ .

12. Events concurrent with the institution of a treatment that can affect the dependent variable constitute the threat of _____ .

13. The group to whom a researcher *ideally* can generalize the research findings is the _____ population.

14. Novelty effects represent a threat to the _____
    _____ validity of a study.

15. When data are collected at a single point in time, the design is referred to as
    _____ .

16. Longitudinal studies conducted to determine the long-term outcome of some
    condition or intervention are called _____
    _____ .

C. Study Questions

1. Define the following terms. Compare your definition with the definition in Chapter 12 of the textbook or in the glossary.

   a. Research design: _____
   _____
   _____

   b. Randomized block design: _____
   _____
   _____

   c. Matching: _____
   _____
   _____

   d. Analysis of covariance: _____
   _____
   _____

   e. Repeated measures design: _____
   _____
   _____

f. Threats to internal validity: _____

_____

_____

g. Selection threat: _____

_____

_____

h. Attrition: _____

_____

_____

i. External validity: _____

_____

_____

j. Accessible population: _____

_____

_____

k. Power: _____

_____

_____

l. Longitudinal study: _____

_____

_____

m. Trend study: _____

_____

_____

n. Panel study: _____

_____

_____

2. Examine the ten problem statements in the matching exercise of Chapter 10. For each, specify one or more extraneous variables that the researcher might want to control.

   1. _____

   2. _____

   3. _____

   4. _____

   5. _____

   6. _____

   7. _____

   8. _____

   9. _____

   10. _____

3. A nurse researcher is interested in comparing the oral and rectal temperature measurements of febrile adults at two times a day on three different wards. Could such a study be conducted as a factorial experiment? Why or why not? If yes, what are the factors in the design? Could this study be conducted as a repeated measures design? Why or why not? If yes, how would you counterbalance? Could a randomized block design be used? Why or why not? If yes, what would the blocking variable be?

4. Suppose you wanted to study the coping strategies of AIDS patients at different points in the progress of the disease. Design a cross-sectional study to research this question, describing how subjects would be selected. Now design a longitudinal study to research the same problem. Identify the strengths and weaknesses of the two approaches.

5. Below is a list of ten target populations. For each, think of an accessible population (i.e., a population accessible to *you*) that you might be able to use if you were conducting the study. Be as specific (and realistic) as possible.

   a. All pregnant women residing in an urban area. _____

   _____

   _____

b. All high school students applying to schools of nursing. _____

_____

_____

c. All parents of children born with spina bifida. _____

_____

_____

d. All faculty teaching psychiatric nursing in universities. _____

_____

_____

e. All cigarette smokers. _____

_____

_____

f. All women using an IUD. _____

_____

_____

g. All men over 45 who have had a cardiovascular accident. _____

_____

_____

h. All licensed midwives. _____

_____

_____

i. All male nurses employed in intensive care units. _____

_____

_____

j. All appendectomy patients hospitalized for seven or more days. _____

_____

_____

6. Below is a schematic diagram representing the variability in a dependent variable, patient satisfaction with nursing care. Draw in some circles representing your hypotheses for variables that affect patient satisfaction. (NOTE: If the variables you identify are *themselves* related to one another, then the circles you draw in should overlap with each other as well with the patient satisfaction circle.)

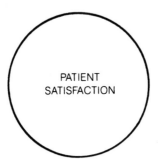

7. Suppose you wanted to study the effect of an experimental approach to teaching student nurses how to give subcutaneous injections. In conducting a true experiment for this study, what environmental factors would you want to control with respect to maintaining constancy of conditions?

D. Application Exercises

Wilkins (1990)* investigated the relationship between the use of IUDs and the incidence of pelvic inflammatory disease (PID) in a sample of urban women. The data were gathered from the gynecology departments of four health centers (one university, one city hospital, one health maintenance organization, and one consortium of private gynecologists). Wilkins obtained the records of 600 women—150 from each facility—who were diagnosed within the previous 12 months as having PID. She also obtained the records of 150 women who had come to each of the facilities for some other purpose and who had no record of having had PID within the 12-month period prior to their focal visit. The two groups of 600 women (the PID and non-PID group) were matched in terms of age (within a five-year age range of under 20, 20–25, 26–29, 30–35, etc.) and marital status (currently married or not married). For each of the 1200 women, the records were examined to determine whether they had had an IUD inserted within two years prior to their focal visit. For those women for whom no determination could be made based on the records of the facility, brief telephone interviews were administered to obtain the needed information (30 women who could not be reached were replaced with other women to maintain the sample

*This example is fictitious.

size). The data revealed that 122 women in the PID group (20.3 percent), compared with 74 women in the non-PID group (12.3 percent), had used an IUD, a significant group difference. Based on this analysis, Wilkins concluded that use of an IUD was a causative factor of PID in this sample.

1. Review and critique this study. Suggest alternative designs for examining the research problem. To assist you in your critique, here are some guiding questions:

   a. Is this research nonexperimental? If so, is it *inherently* nonexperimental? Why or why not?

   b. Evaluate the internal validity of the study. What threats to its internal validity, if any, are posed?

   c. Examine the criteria for causality presented in Chapter 9 of the text. Does this study meet all of the criteria for establishing causality?

   d. The researcher concluded that her independent variable (use of the IUD) "caused" certain outcomes (incidence of PID). Can you offer two or more alternative explanations to account for the outcome?

   e. What extraneous variables did the researcher identify, and by what method were they controlled? How else might those variables have been controlled?

   f. What extraneous variables do you think *should* have been controlled but were not? Why might the researcher have decided *not* to control these variables?

   g. To what extent did the researcher control for the constancy of conditions in this study? Suggest ways in which this aspect of the study could have been improved.

   h. What is the target population of this study? What is the accessible population? How reasonable is it to generalize the results of this study to the target population?

   i. Evaluate the external validity of the study in terms of the "threats" described in Chapter 12. What changes, if any, would you recommend to improve the external validity of the design?

2. Below are several suggested research articles. Read one or more of these articles and respond to questions a–i of Question D.1 in terms of these actual research studies.

   • Beckman, C.A. (1990). Postterm pregnancy: Effects on temperature and glucose regulation. *Nursing Research, 39,* 21–24.

   • Buckwalter, K.C., Cusack, D., Sidles, E., Wadle, K., and Beaver, M. (1989). Increasing communication ability in aphasic/dysarthric patients. *Western Journal of Nursing Research, 11,* 736–747.

   • Fridh, G., Kopare, T., Gaston-Johansson, F., and Norvell, K., (1988). Factors associated with more intense labor pain. *Research in Nursing and Health, 11,* 117–124.

   • Gennaro, S. (1988). Postpartal anxiety and depression in mothers of term and preterm infants. *Nursing Research, 37,* 82–89.

- Giuffre, M., Heidenreich, T., Carney-Gersten, P., Dorsch, J.A., and Heidenreich, E. (1990). The relationship between axillary and core body temperature measurements. *Applied Nursing Research, 3*, 52–55.

Wyland (1990)* hypothesized that aging negatively affects intellectual capacity and motor responsivity. To test this hypothesis, she randomly selected the names of 250 men aged 70 or above; 250 men in their 50s; and 250 men in their 30s from the residents living in a mid-sized city in Illinois. Wyland realized that intellectual capacity is sometimes correlated with social class. Furthermore, mortality rates vary by social class. Therefore, the subjects were selected in such a way that half in each group were from lower-income households (household incomes $20,000 or less) and half were from higher-income households (income over $20,000). The basic design for the analysis, therefore, was as follows:

	Age Group		
Income Group	30s	50s	70s
≤ $20,000			
> $20,000			

The 750 individuals were administered an individual intelligence test that measured verbal aptitude, problem solving, quantitative skills, spatial aptitude, and overall intelligence. In addition, the participants were given various reaction-time tests. The analysis of the data revealed that, as hypothesized, intelligence declined with age in both income groups. Except on the measure of verbal aptitude, the subjects in their 30s scored highest, and the subjects in their 70s scored lowest on the subtests of intellectual capacity and on overall intelligence. The same pattern was observed for reaction time. Wyland concluded that the aging process causes deterioration of both intellectual and motor capacity.

3. Review and critique Wyland's study. Suggest alternative designs or other modifications for testing the researcher's hypothesis. Use questions a through i from Exercise D.1, above, to guide you in your critique. In addition, answer the following questions:

   a. Is this design cross-sectional or longitudinal?

   b. What problems, if any, does this design pose in terms of testing the hypothesis?

   c. What design, if any, might be more appropriate?

   d. What difficulties, if any, would the researcher have had in implementing your recommended design?

*This example is fictitious.

4. Below are several suggested research articles. Read the introductory and methods sections of one or more of these articles and respond to the questions in Exercise D.3 in terms of these actual research studies.

- Harrison, T. M., Pistolessi, T. U., and Stephen, T. D. (1989). Assessing nurses' communication style. *Western Journal of Nursing Research, 11*, 75–91.
- Mendelson, M. A., Skinner, R. A., and Proctor, M. B. (1985). Attitudes toward a social issue in health care: A cohort analysis. *Research in Nursing and Health, 8*, 307–312.
- Mercer, R. T., and Ferketich, S. L. (1990). Predictors of family functioning eight months following birth. *Nursing Research, 39*, 76–82.
- Tulman, L., Fawcett, J., Groblewski, L. and Silverman, L. (1990). Changes in functional status after childbirth. *Nursing Research, 39*, 70–75.

E. Special Projects

1. Suppose that you wanted to compare premature and normal babies in terms of their development at age five. Describe how you would design such a study, being careful to indicate what extraneous variables you would need to control and how you would control them.

2. A nurse researcher is interested in testing the effect of packing sugar on a wound on the wound-healing process. Describe a design you would recommend for this problem, being careful to indicate what extraneous variables you would need to control and how you would control them.

3. Chapter 12 identified four types of situations in which it might be appropriate to use multiple points of data collection. Develop a researchable problem statement for each of these four situations. Develop a design for studying one or more of these problems.

   a. Time-related phenomena: _____

   _____

   _____

   b. Time-sequenced phenomena: _____

   _____

   _____

   c. Comparative purposes: _____

   _____

   _____

   d. Enhancement of internal validity: _____

   _____

   _____

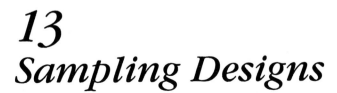

13
Sampling Designs

A. Matching Exercises

Match each statement relating to sampling from Set B with one of the phrases from Set A. Indicate the letter corresponding to your response next to each of the statements in Set B.

SET A
a. Probability sampling
b. Nonprobability sampling
c. Both probability and nonprobability sampling
d. Neither probability nor nonprobability sampling

SET B	**RESPONSE**
1. Includes systematic sampling	_____
2. Allows an estimation of the magnitude of sampling error	_____
3. Guarantees a representative sample	_____
4. Includes quota sampling	_____
5. Yields better results when the samples are large	_____
6. Elements are selected by nonrandom methods	_____
7. Can be used with entire populations or with selected strata from the populations	_____
8. Used to select populations	_____
9. Provides an equal chance of elements being selected	_____
10. Is required when the population is homogeneous	_____

B. Completion Exercises

Write the words or phrases that correctly complete the sentences below.

1. A(n) _____
   is a subset of the units that comprise the population.

2. The main criterion for evaluating a sample is its _____

   _____ .

3. A sample would be considered _____

   _____

   if it systematically overrepresented or underrepresented a segment of the population.

4. If a population is completely _____

   _____

   with respect to key attributes, then any sample is as good as any other.

5. Another term used for convenience sample is _____

   _____ .

6. Quota samples are essentially accidental samples from selected _____

   _____ of the population.

7. Another term for a purposive sample is a(n) _____

   _____ sample.

8. The most basic type of probability sampling is referred to as _____

   _____ .

9. When disproportional sampling is used, an adjustment procedure known as

   _____

   is normally used to estimate population values.

10. Another term used to refer to cluster sampling is _____

    _____ sampling.

11. In systematic samples, the distance between selected elements is referred to as the

    _____

    _____ .

12. Differences between population values and sample values are referred to as the

    _____ .

13. If a researcher has confidence in his or her sampling design, the results of a study can reasonably be generalized to the _____ population.

14. As a sample _____ , the probability of drawing a deviant sample diminishes.

15. If a researcher wanted to draw a systematic sample of 100 from a population of 3000, the sampling interval would be _____ .

C. Study Questions

1. Define the following terms. Compare your definition with the definition in Chapter 13 of the textbook or in the glossary.

   a. Sampling: _____

   _____

   _____

   b. Elements: _____

   _____

   _____

   c. Probability sampling: _____

   _____

   _____

   d. Nonprobability sampling: _____

   _____

   _____

   e. Stratum: _____

   _____

   _____

   f. Eligibility criteria: _____

   _____

   _____

g. Convenience sample: _____

_____

_____

h. Snowball sampling: _____

_____

_____

i. Quota sample: _____

_____

_____

j. Purposive sample: _____

_____

_____

k. Random sample: _____

_____

_____

l. Sampling frame: _____

_____

_____

m. Stratified random sampling: _____

_____

_____

n. Disproportional sampling design: _____

_____

_____

o. Cluster sampling: _____

_____

_____

p. Systematic sampling: _____

_____

_____

2. Using the table of random numbers presented in Table 9.1, select a random sample of 30 names, drawn from a sampling frame of your choice (e.g., a page from a telephone directory, roster of nursing students, a staff list, etc.).

3. For each of the following target populations, identify an accessible population (accessible to *you*) that might be used in a study.

TARGET POPULATION   **ACCESSIBLE POPULATION**

a. All teenagers diagnosed as having
   scoliosis in the U.S.   a. _____

b. All nursing home residents over
   the age of 70 in the U.S.   b. _____

c. All persons eligible to receive   c. _____
   Medicaid

d. All rape victims in the U.S.   d. _____

e. All persons with blood type O
   positive   e. _____

4. Identify the type of sampling design used in the following examples:

                                                   TYPE OF DESIGN

a. Thirty nursing faculty randomly
   sampled from a random selection
   of ten nursing schools   _____

b. All the nurses participating in a
   continuing education seminar   _____

c. A sample of 250 members randomly selected from a roster of
   ANA members   _____

d. Every 20th patient admitted to the
   emergency room in the month of
   June   _____

e. The first 20 male and the first 20
   female patients admitted to the
   hospital with hypothermia   _____

5. Nurse A is planning to study the effects of maternal stress, maternal depression, maternal age, family economic resources, and social support on a child's socioemotional development among both intact and mother-headed families. Nurse

B is planning to study body position on patients' respiratory functioning. Describe the kinds of samples that the two nurses would need to use. Which nurse would need the larger sample? Defend your answer.

D. Application Exercises

Layden (1991)* studied the job-search strategies of recent nursing school graduates. Her survey focused on such issues as timing of job applications, number of applications, source of information about jobs, method of initial contact, and so on. She was interested in learning whether certain strategies were more successful in achieving job offers (and acceptable job offers) than others. She obtained lists of graduates from six schools of nursing in Greater Boston (two schools for each of three different types of programs). She then conducted telephone interviews with 100 graduates from each of the three program types (Bachelors, diploma, and Associates). Her method was to find, using local telephone directories, the telephone numbers for as many of the names on her lists as she could and to make calls until she had completed 100 interviews with graduates from each group. Thus, her final sample consisted of 300 recently graduated RNs.

1. Review and critique this research effort. Suggest alternative sampling designs. To assist you in your critique, here are some guiding questions:
   a. What type of sampling design was used? Was this design appropriate? Would you recommend a different sampling approach? Why or why not? What are the advantages of the approach used? What are the disadvantages?
   b. Identify what you believe to be the target and accessible populations in this study. How representative do you feel the accessible population is of the target population? How representative is the sample of this accessible population? What are some of the possible sources of sampling bias?
   c. Did the researcher use a proportional or disproportional sampling plan? Is this appropriate? Why or why not?
   d. Comment on the size of the sample. Does this sample size appear to be adequate?

2. Below are several suggested research articles. Read the introductory and methods sections of one or more of these articles and respond to questions a through d of Exercise D.1 in terms of these actual research studies.

   • Brown, B., Roberts, J., Browne, G., Byrne, C., Love, B., and Streiner, D. (1988). Gender differences in variables associated with psychosocial adjustment to a burn injury. *Research in Nursing and Health, 11,* 23–30.

*This example is fictitious.

- Engel, N.S. (1987). Menopausal stage, current life change, attitude toward women's roles, and perceived health status. *Nursing Research, 36,* 353–357.
- Lierman, L.M., Young, H.M., Kasprzyk, D., and Benoliel, J. (1990). Predicting breast self-examination using the theory of reasoned action. *Nursing Research, 39,* 97–101.
- Lookinland, S. (1989). Comparison of pulmonary vascular pressure based on blood volume and ventilator status. *Nursing Research, 38,* 68–71.
- Rustia, J. and Abbott, D.A. (1990). Predicting paternal role enactment. *Western Journal of Nursing Research, 12,* 145–160.

E. Special Projects

1. Suppose that you were interested in studying preventive health-care behaviors among low-income urban residents. Describe how you might select a sample for your study using the following:

   a. A convenience sample

   b. A quota sample

   c. A cluster sample

2. Propose a researchable problem statement. Specify a research and sampling design to study this problem. In particular, specify the following:

   - The target population, including all criteria for inclusion in the population
   - An accessible population
   - A sampling design, together with a rationale
   - A recommended sample size

   With respect to the latter three aspects, be realistic. Take into account your resources, time, and level of expertise. That is, recommend a plan that would be feasible to implement.

Part IV

Measurement and Data Collection

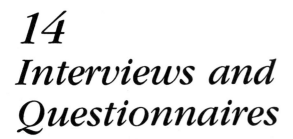

14
Interviews and Questionnaires

A. Matching Exercises

Match each descriptive statement regarding self-report methods from Set B with one of the statements from Set A. Indicate the letter corresponding to your response next to each item in Set B.

SET A
a. An interview schedule
b. A questionnaire
c. Both an interview schedule and a questionnaire
d. Neither an interview schedule nor a questionnaire

SET B   **RESPONSE**

1. Can provide respondents the protection of anonymity   _____
2. Can be used with illiterate respondents   _____
3. Can contain both open- and closed-ended questions   _____
4. Is used in survey research   _____
5. Is the best way to measure human behavior   _____
6. Generally yields high response rates   _____
7. Can control the order in which questions are asked and answered   _____
8. Is generally an inexpensive method of data collection   _____

9. Requires that the purpose of the study be unknown to the subject   _____

10. Benefits from pretesting   _____

B. Completion Exercises

Write the words or phrases that correctly complete the sentences below.

1. The four dimensions along which data collection methods can vary are _____

   _____ , _____ ,

   _____ , and _____ .

2. Subjects in self-report studies are often referred to as _____

   _____ .

3. In a focused interview, general question areas are normally prepared in the form

   of a _____ .

4. When a group of respondents is assembled in one place to discuss questions simultaneously, the approach being used is often referred to as a _____

   _____ .

5. The approach used to question people about important events, decisions, or turning points is referred to as _____

   _____ .

6. A disadvantage of _____ questions is that the researcher may inadvertently omit some potentially important alternatives.

7. _____ questions are relatively inefficient in terms of the respondents' time.

8. If respondents are not very verbal or articulate _____

   _____ questions are generally most appropriate.

9. The type of instrument that typically uses more closed-ended than open-ended questions is the _____

   _____ .

10. Response alternatives should be mutually _____ .

11. Questions that require respondents to select between two alternatives are known

    as _____

    _____ items.

12. Another term for two-dimensional checklists is _____ _____ .

13. Interviewer probes should always be _____ _____ .

14. Respondents are less likely to give "don't know" responses in a(n) _____ _____ situation.

15. Nonresponse in self-report studies is generally not _____ _____ and can therefore lead to bias.

C. Study Questions

1. Define the following terms. Compare your definition with the definition in Chapter 14 of the textbook or in the glossary.

   a. Unstructured interview: _____

   _____

   _____

   b. Focused interview: _____

   _____

   _____

   c. Life history: _____

   _____

   _____

   d. Interview schedule: _____

   _____

   _____

   e. Questionnaire: _____

   _____

   _____

f. Open-ended questions: _____

_____

_____

g. Fixed-alternative questions: _____

_____

_____

h. Cover letter: _____

_____

_____

i. Dichotomous items: _____

_____

_____

j. "Cafeteria" question: _____

_____

_____

k. Matrix question: _____

_____

_____

l. Module: _____

_____

_____

m. Pretest: _____

_____

_____

n. Follow-up reminder: _____

_____

_____

o. Probe: _____

_____

_____

p. Response rate: _____

_____

_____

2. Below are several research problems. Indicate which type of unstructured approach you might recommend using for each. Defend your response.

a. By what process do parents of a handicapped child learn to cope with their

child's problem? _____

_____

b. What are the barriers to preventive health care practices among the urban

poor? _____

_____

_____

c. What stresses does the spouse of a terminally ill patient experience? _____

_____

d. What type of information does a nurse draw on most heavily in formulating

nursing diagnoses? _____

_____

e. What are the coping mechanisms and perceived barriers to coping among

severely disfigured burn patients? _____

_____

_____

3. Suppose you were interested in studying the barriers that low-income women experience in obtaining adequate routine health care for themselves and their children. Develop a topic guide for a focused interview on this topic.

4. For the study described in Question 3, develop ten closed-ended questions.

5. Compare the nature of the information you would obtain for the research prob-

lem described in Question 3 using the topic guide versus using the closed-ended questions. Which approach would yield more useful information? Defend your response.

6. Suppose you were interested in studying nurses' attitudes toward "surrogate mothers." Develop the following types of questions designed to measure these attitudes.

    a. Dichotomous item: _____

    _____

    _____

    b. Multiple choice item: _____

    _____

    _____

    c. Open-ended item: _____

    _____

    _____

7. Suggest response alternatives for the following questions that might appear in a questionnaire.
    a. In a typical month, how frequently do you have sexual intercourse?
    b. When was the last time you had your blood pressure tested?
    c. Which of the following statements best describes your attitudes towards nurse practitioners?
    d. What is your marital status?
    e. How would you rate your nursing research instruction in terms of overall quality of teaching?
    f. How often do you skip breakfast?
    g. How important is it to you to avoid a pregnancy at this time?
    h. How many cigarettes do you smoke in a typical day?
    i. From which of the following sources have you learned about the dangers of smoking?
    j. Which of the following statements best describes the physical pain you experienced during labor and delivery?

8. Read the following article and describe the data collection instruments in terms of

the four dimensions discussed in this chapter: structure, quantifiability, researcher obtrusiveness, and objectivity:

• Mangelsdorf, K.R. and Smith, H.L. (1990). Toward a cross-cultural view of job satisfaction in nursing. *Western Journal of Nursing Research*, *12*, 386–401.

D. Application Exercises

Holle (1990)* conducted a survey that focused on drug usage patterns in an urban adolescent population. The survey used self-administered questionnaires that were distributed to 25 high schools and administered in group (home room) sessions to 3,568 respondents. The questionnaire consisted of 56 closed-ended and two open-ended questions. Included were background questions; questions on the students' attitudes toward, knowledge of, and experience with various drugs; and questions on the students' physical and mental health. The instrument was pretested with ten college freshmen prior to administration.

1. Review and critique the above description of the overall study. Suggest possible alternative ways of collecting the data for the research problem. To assist you in your critique, here are some guiding questions:

   a. The data in this study were collected by self-report. Could the data have been collected in another way? *Should* they have been, in your opinion?

   b. Were the data collected by questionnaire or interview? Was the decision to use this method appropriate or would you recommend an alternative procedure? Comment on the advantages and disadvantages of the procedure used for this particular research problem.

   c. Comment on the degree of structure of the instrument used. Would you recommend a more structured or a less structured instrument? Why or why not?

   d. Was the instrument adequately pretested?

   e. Comment on the method in which the instrument was administered. Was the method efficient? Did it yield an adequate response rate? Did it appear costly? What opportunity did respondents have to obtain clarifying information about the questions?

2. Below are several suggested research articles. Skim one or more of these articles, paying particular attention to the methods used to measure research variables and collect the data. Then respond to questions a to e from Question D.1 in terms of this actual research study.

*This example is fictitious.

- Gillett, P.A. (1988). Self-reported factors influencing exercise adherence in over-weight women. *Nursing Research, 37*, 25–29.
- Kearnery, M.H., Cronenwett, L.R., and Barrett, J.A. (1990). Breast-feeding problems in the first week postpartum. *Nursing Research, 39*, 90–95.
- Nettles-Carlson, B., Field, M.L., Friedman, B.J. and Smith, L.S. (1988). Effectiveness of teaching breast self-examination during office visits. *Research in Nursing and Health, 11*, 41–50.
- Norberg, A. and Asplund, K. (1990). Caregivers' experience of caring for severely demented patients. *Western Journal of Nursing Research, 12*, 75–84.

3. Holle, in her study of drug use patterns among high school students, accompanied each questionnaire with the following cover letter:

Dear Student:

This questionnaire is part of a study to learn about some health-related issues among high school students. Through this study we hope to have a better understanding of young people in America. Students from 25 high schools in the United States are being asked to help us in this effort. Your high school was selected at random.

Your responses to this questionnaire are completely anonymous. No one will know your answers. So, even though some of the questions are very personal, we hope that you will answer honestly. The quality of the picture we will have of high school students today depends upon your willingness to provide thorough and honest answers.

Please answer every question. When you are through, please turn the questionnaire in to your home room teacher.

Your cooperation in completing this questionnaire is deeply appreciated.

Sincerely,
Paula Holle, R.N.

Review and critique this sample cover letter. Analyze the tone, wording, and content of the letter. Compare the content with the suggested contents of such a letter presented in Chapter 14 of the textbook.

E. Special Projects

1. Develop a short (2–3 pages) questionnaire, properly formatted and sequenced, for a study of nurses' experiences with victims of child abuse.
2. Draft a cover letter to accompany the instrument developed in Exercise E.1.

3. Suggest one open-ended and one closed-ended question relating to each of the following variables. Compare the quality and amount of information that could be obtained with each.

    a. Women's attitudes toward nurse–midwives
    b. Factors influencing a decision to obtain a vasectomy
    c. Perceived adequacy of community health-care services
    d. Student nurses' first experiences with the death of a patient
    e. Factors influencing nurses' administration of pain-relieving narcotics to patients

4. Develop a topic guide that focuses on nursing students' reasons for selecting nursing as a career, and their satisfactions and dissatisfactions with their decision. Administer the topic guide to five first-year nursing students in a face-to-face interview situation. Now administer the topic guide in a focus group setting with five nursing students. Compare the kinds of information that the two approaches yield. What, if anything, did you learn in the group setting that did not emerge in the personal interviews (and vice versa)?

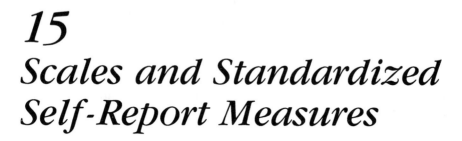

15
Scales and Standardized Self-Report Measures

A. Matching Exercises

Match each descriptive statement from Set B with one (or more) of the statements from Set A. Indicate the letter(s) corresponding to your response next to each item in Set B.

SET A
a. Likert scales
b. Guttman scales
c. Semantic differential scales
d. None of the above (a–c)

SET B   **RESPONSE**

1. Does not permit fine discriminations among respondents   _____
2. Can be used to measure attitudes   _____
3. Is sometimes referred to as a summated rating scale   _____
4. Is subject to response set biases   _____
5. Is often used to measure behavioral characteristics   _____
6. Presents statements to which respondents indicate agreement
   or disagreement   _____
7. Rarely contains more than five items   _____
8. Uses a graphic rating scale format   _____

9. Reversal of items plays a role in minimizing response set biases such as acquiescence _____

10. Provides a quantitative measure of an attribute _____

B. Completion Exercises

Write the words or phrases that correctly complete the sentences below.

1. Scales are designed to measure _____

_____

of an attribute a person or object possesses.

2. Likert scales consist of a number of statements written in the _____

_____ form.

3. Some people omit the category labelled _____

_____ in constructing Likert scales, to avoid "fence-sitting."

4. In Likert scales, positively worded statements are scored in one direction, and the scoring of negatively worded statements is _____

_____ .

5. In Likert scales, statements that are endorsed or rejected by most respondents should be _____

_____ .

6. Another term used to refer to Guttman scales is _____

_____ .

7. The procedure for determining the unidimensionality of Guttman scales is referred to as _____

_____ .

8. Semantic differentials tend to yield measures of _____

_____ independent dimensions.

9. For the measurement of attitudes, the dimension referred to as _____

_____ on semantic differentials is most useful.

10. The bias introduced when respondents select options at either end of the response continuum is known as _____

_____ .

C. Study Questions

1. Define the following terms. Compare your definition with the definition in Chapter 15 of the textbook or in the glossary.

   a. Scale: _____

   _____

   _____

   b. Likert scale: _____

   _____

   _____

   c. Guttman scale: _____

   _____

   _____

   d. Reproducibility: _____

   _____

   _____

   e. Semantic differential: _____

   _____

   _____

   f. Response sets: _____

   _____

   _____

   g. Social desirability response set: _____

   _____

   _____

   h. Acquiescence response set: _____

   _____

   _____

   i. "Nay-sayer": _____

   _____

   _____

j. Visual analogue scale: _____

_____

_____

2. Below are hypothetical responses for Respondent Y and Respondent Z to the Likert statements presented in Table 15.1 of the textbook. What would the total score for both of these respondents be, using the scoring rules described in Chapter 15?

ITEM NO.	RESPONDENT Y	RESPONDENT Z
1	D	SA
2	A	D
3	SA	D
4	?	A
5	D	SA
6	SA	D
7	A	SD
8	SA	D
9	D	?
10	SD	A
Total score:	_____	_____

3. Below are hypothetical responses for Respondents A, B, C, and D to the Likert statements presented in Table 15.1 of the text. Three of these four sets of responses contain some indication of a possible response set bias. Identify *which* three, and identify the types of bias.

ITEM NO.	RESPONDENT A	RESPONDENT B	RESPONDENT C	RESPONDENT D
1	A	SA	SD	D
2	A	SD	SA	SD
3	SA	D	SA	D
4	A	A	SD	SD
5	?	A	SD	SD
6	A	D	SA	D
7	SA	SD	SA	D
8	A	D	SA	?
9	A	A	SD	?
10	SA	?	SD	D
Bias:	_____	_____	_____	_____

4. Below are ten attitudinal statements regarding attitudes toward natural family planning. For each statement, indicate how you think the item would be scored (i.e., would "strongly agree" be assigned a score of 1 or 5, assuming high scores reflect more favorable attitudes)? What is the maximum and minimum score possible on this scale?

STATEMENT   **SCORE FOR "STRONGLY AGREE"**

a. Natural family planning is an effective method of avoiding unwanted
   pregnancies.   _____

b. Natural family planning removes
   the spontaneity from lovemaking.   _____

c. Using natural family planning
   methods is too time-consuming.   _____

d. A man and a woman can be drawn
   closer together by collaborating in
   using natural family planning.   _____

e. Natural family planning is the saf-
   est form of birth control.   _____

f. Natural family planning is too risky
   if one really doesn't want a
   pregnancy.   _____

g. Natural family planning puts a
   woman in better touch with her
   body.   _____

h. Natural family planning is an acceptable form of contraception.   _____

i. All in all, natural family planning is
   the best method of birth control.   _____

j. Natural family planning is "un-
   natural" in terms of the restrictions
   it imposes on lovemaking.   _____

5. Select items from Exercise C.4, above, that might be used to construct a Guttman scale. Test whether your suggested scale works by asking friends to respond and then trying to reproduce their scores.

6. Identify five constructs of clinical relevance that would be appropriate for measurement using a visual analogue scale (VAS).

D. Application Exercises

Kestacher (1990)* wanted to conduct a survey of nurses' attitudes toward abortion. For this study she prepared 20 statements pro and con. After developing the items, she asked ten of her colleagues to indicate their level of agreement or

*This example is fictitious.

disagreement with the statements, on a seven-point scale. Kestacher used the data from these ten nurses as pretest data for refining the instrument. The original 20 items are presented below:

1. Every woman has a right to obtain an abortion if she does not want a baby.
2. Abortion should be made available to women on demand.
†3. The government should subsidize the cost of abortions for poor women.
4. Abortions should be made illegal.
5. The right to an abortion should be available to all women.
†6. Women whose lives are in danger because of their pregnancy should be allowed to have an abortion.
7. Abortion is morally wrong.
8. Women need to have control of their own bodies by having abortion services available to them.
9. Women who have abortions are murderers.
10. People who oppose abortions have no compassion for women's circumstances.
11. Legalizing abortion is a sign of the decay of civilization.
12. No decent woman would even consider killing her own baby through abortion.
13. The freedom to choose an abortion is essential to the liberation of women.
14. An enlightened society gives its citizens the right to make important choices, such as having an abortion.
15. The right to obtain a legal abortion should never be denied to women.
16. Women who have abortions demonstrate the courage to make a tough decision.
17. No woman should be forced to bear a baby she does not want.
†18. If men had to bear babies, abortions would never have been illegal.
19. Abortion is one of the most despicable acts that a human can commit.
20. Women should have the right to choose having an abortion.

Upon reviewing the pretest responses, Kestacher eliminated items 3, 6, and 18 (indicated with a dagger). She then had a 17-item scale ready to use in her survey.

1. Read and critique the description of Kestacher's activities. Suggest possible alternative ways of collecting the data for the research problem. To assist you in your critique, here are some guiding questions:

   a. What type of scale did the researcher develop? Was this type of scale best suited to the needs of the researcher, or would another type of scale have been more appropriate? Why or why not?

   b. Given the aims of the researcher, was the development of *any* type of scale appropriate? That is, could the data have been collected by another method? *Should* they have been, in your opinion?

   c. Comment on the procedures used by the researcher to develop the scale. Was the scale adequately reviewed and pretested?

d. Critique the quality of the scale itself. Does it consist of a sufficient number of items? Is the number of response alternatives good? Does the scale do an adequate job of minimizing bias? If not, suggest modifications that might reduce response set biases.

e. Do you think the scale is unidimensional? That is, does it appear to be measuring one (and only one) underlying concept?

f. Comment on why you think the items that were eliminated (items 3, 6, and 18) were removed from the final scale.

g. Do you feel the researcher needed to develop this scale from scratch?

2. Below are several suggested research articles in which one or more scales was used. Review one or more of the articles and respond to questions a to g from Question D.1, to the extent possible, in terms of this study. (N.B.: The more technical aspects of the studies should just be briefly skimmed for the present exercise.)

- Brown, M.S. and Tanner, C. (1990). Measurement of Type A behavior in pre-schoolers. *Nursing Research, 39,* 207–211.
- Godschalx, S.M. (1984). Effect of a mental health educational program upon police officers. *Research in Nursing and Health, 7,* 111–117.
- LaMonica, E.L., Oberst, M.T., Madea, A.R., and Wolf, R.M. (1986). Development of a patient satisfaction scale. *Research in Nursing and Health, 9,* 43–50.
- Morgan, B.S. (1984). A semantic differential measure of attitudes toward black American patients. *Research in Nursing and Health, 7,* 155–162.

E. Special Projects

1. Develop semantic differential scales to measure attitudes toward the following concepts: cancer, heart attack, kidney failure, and brain damage.

2. Describe a potential use for the semantic differential scales described in Exercise E.1, above. What kind of comparisons might you make in such a study?

3. Suppose that you were interested in studying nurse's attitudes toward AIDS patients. Develop five positively worded and five negatively worded statements that could be used to construct a Likert scale for such a study.

4. Construct a VAS to measure fatigue. Administer the VAS two ways: (1) to yourself at 10 different times of the day; and (2) to ten different people at the same time of day. For the two types of administrations, is there similarity in scores, or is there a wide range of responses? Which of the two yields scores with a wider range?

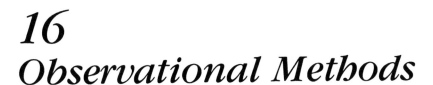

16
Observational Methods

A. Matching Exercises

Match each problem statement from Set B with one of the statements from Set A. Indicate the letter corresponding to your response next to each item in Set B.

SET A
a. The study would *require* observational data.
b. The study *could* use observational data, as well as other forms of data.
c. The study is not amenable to observational data collection.

SET B	RESPONSE
1. Are nurses' attitudes toward abortion related to their years of nursing experience?	_____
2. Are patients' levels of stress related to their willingness to disclose their own fears to nursing staff?	_____
3. Are the sleep–wake patterns of infants related to their gestational age at birth?	_____
4. Is the degree of physical activity of a psychiatric patient related to his or her length of hospitalization?	_____
5. Are nurses' licensure examination scores more highly related to their clinical grades or to their grades in academic courses?	_____
6. Is a child's fear during immunization related to the nurse's method of preparing the child for the shot?	_____

7. Does the presence of the father in the delivery room affect the mother's level of pain? _____

8. Is the ability of dialysis patients to cleanse and dress their shunts related to their self-esteem and locus of control? _____

9. Is the level of achievement motivation among nursing students related to their clinical speciality? _____

10. Is aggressive behavior among hospitalized mentally retarded children related to styles of discipline by hospital staff? _____

B. Completion Exercises

Write the words or phrases that correctly complete the sentences below.

1. The major focus of observation in nursing research is the _____ _____ and _____ of humans.

2. When the unit of observation is small, specific behaviors, the approach is said to be _____ _____.

3. The reactive measurement effect may occur when the observer is _____ _____.

4. The sociological technique known as _____ _____ involves the collection of unstructured observational data.

5. The fourth phase of a participant observer's role involves _____ _____.

6. The three major types of observational positioning in participant observation studies are _____ , _____ , and _____ positioning.

7. The four types of field notes are _____ , _____ , _____ , and _____ notes.

8. In a structured observational setting, the most common procedure is to construct a(n) _____

_____ for observed behaviors.

9. In general, less observer inference is required when the units of behavior being observed are _____

_____ .

10. _____ is the method of obtaining representative observations without observing all behaviors or activities of interest.

11. Observers need to be carefully _____

in the use of a structured observational instrument.

12. One of the major difficulties with observational data is the possibility that the data are not _____

_____ .

13. The tendency for observers to rate things too positively is a bias known as the

_____ .

14. An observer bias in which extreme events are given mid-range ratings is known as a bias toward _____

_____ .

15. The tendency for observers to rate things too negatively is a bias known as the

_____ .

C. Study Questions

1. Define the following terms. Compare your definition with the definition in Chapter 16 of the textbook or in the glossary.

   a. Molar unit of analysis: _____

   _____

   _____

   b. Reactivity: _____

   _____

   _____

   c. Participant observation: _____

_____

_____

   d. Log: _____

_____

_____

   e. Multiple positioning: _____

_____

_____

   f. Mobile positioning: _____

_____

_____

   g. Field notes: _____

_____

_____

   h. Checklist: _____

_____

_____

   i. Sign system: _____

_____

_____

   j. Rating scale: _____

_____

_____

   k. Time sampling: _____

_____

_____

   l. Event sampling: _____

_____

_____

m. Interrater reliability: _____

_____

_____

n. Central tendency bias: _____

_____

_____

o. Enhancement of contrast bias: _____

_____

_____

p. Halo effect: _____

_____

_____

2. Below are ten problem statements in which the dependent variable of interest is amenable to observation. Indicate your recommendation for the relationship between the observer and subjects along the concealment/intervention dimensions for each problem. Justify your response.

a. What is the effect of touch on the crying behavior of hospitalized children?

_____

_____

b. What is the effect of increased patient:staff ratios in psychiatric hospitals on interpersonal conflict among staff members?

_____

_____

c. Is the management of appetite loss in burn patients affected by nutritional information provided by nurses?

_____

_____

d. Is the amount and type of information transmitted at the change of shift report affected by the number of years of experience of the nurses?

_____

_____

e. Does a patient's need for personal space vary as a function of age?

_____

_____

f. Are the self-grooming activities of nursing home patients related to the frequency of visits from friends and relatives?

_____

_____

g. Is the adequacy of a student nurse's hand-washing related to his or her type of educational preparation?

_____

_____

h. What is the process by which very low birthweight infants develop the sucking response?

_____

_____

i. What type of patient behaviors are most likely to elicit empathic behaviors in nurses?

_____

_____

j. Do nurses reinforce passive behaviors among female patients more than among male patients?

_____

_____

3. For each of the problem statements indicated above in Exercise C.2, specify whether you think a structured or unstructured approach would be preferable. Justify your response.

a. _____

_____

b. _____

_____

c. _____

_____

d. _____

_____

e. _____

_____

f. _____

_____

g. _____

_____

h. _____

_____

i. _____

_____

j. _____

_____

4. For each of the problem statements listed above in Exercise C.2, indicate whether you think time sampling or event sampling would be preferable. Justify your response.

a. _____

b. _____

c. _____

d. _____

e. _____

f. _____

g. _____

h. _____

i. _____

j. _____

5. Suppose that you were interested in studying verbal interactions among nursing faculty with respect to expressions of solidarity versus antagonism. Would you recommend a molecular unit of analysis (e.g., individual words) or a more molar unit of analysis (e.g., sentences or entire dialogues from staff meetings)? Justify your response.

D. *Application Exercises*

Shehee (1991)* studied the effect of a school nutritional program on the snacking behaviors of students in grades 1 through 6. During the month of October, the experimental program (which consisted of discussion groups led by the school nurse, posters, and classroom activities initiated by the teachers) was introduced into two elementary schools in a large eastern city. Two other schools were used as the controls. The children in all four schools were observed with respect to their selection of snack foods, offered once a week at a 2:00 PM "snack break." Each snack selected was rated in terms of its nutritional value on a scale from 1 to 9. The observations were made by the school nurses who were in the classrooms and noted the selection of each student. Similar observations were made during the months of October (when the program was implemented) and November (after the program was completed). The data consisted of two main types of information: (1) the frequency with which each snack item was selected each week; and (2) the nutritional ratings for the selected snacks for each child. An analysis of these data revealed that the children in the experimental classrooms selected significantly fewer snacks categorized as "nonnutritional salty snacks" (e.g., potato chips) and had a significantly higher average nutritional rating in November than children in the comparison classrooms.

1. Review and critique this study. Suggest alternative ways of collecting the data for the research problem. To assist you in your critique, here are some guiding questions:

    a. The data in this study were collected by observation. Could the data have been collected in another way? *Should* they have been, in your opinion?

    b. Specify the relationship between the observer and those being observed on the concealment and intervention dimensions. Do you feel that the specified relationship is appropriate? What kinds of problems might it raise?

    c. In terms of the unit of observation, would you describe the approach as basically molar or molecular? Do you feel that the level of observation is appropriate, or would you recommend an approach that is more molar or more molecular?

    d. Would you classify the study as having used an unstructured or structured observational procedure? Was the amount of structure in the data collection appropriate, or should there have been more or less structure?

    e. Was the specific procedure used to measure the study variables an adequate way to operationalize the variables? Could you recommend any improvements?

    f. What type of sampling plan was used to sample observations in this study? Would an alternative sampling plan have been better? Why or why not?

*This example is fictitious.

g. What types of observational bias do you think might be operational in this study?

h. Comment on the appropriateness of the persons who made the observations. Can you identify any potential problems with respect to the internal and external validity of the study?

2. Below are several suggested research articles in which an observational approach was used. Review one of the articles and respond to questions a to h from Question D.1, to the extent possible, in terms of this study.

- Fagan, M. J. (1988). Relationship between nurses' assessments of perfusion and toe temperature in pediatric patients with cardiovascular disease. *Heart and Lung, 17*, 157–165.
- Fegley, B. J. (1988). Preparing children for radiologic procedures: Contingent versus noncontingent instruction. *Research in Nursing and Health, 11*, 3–9.
- Harrison, M. J. (1990). A comparison of parental interactions with term and preterm infants. *Research in Nursing and Health, 13*, 173–179.
- Keefe, M. R. (1988). Comparison of neonatal nighttime sleep-wake patterns in nursery versus rooming-in environments. *Nursing Research, 36*, 140–144.
- Whall, A. I., Booth, D. E., Kosinski, J., Donbronski, D., Zakul-Krupa, I. and Weissfield, L. A. (1989). Tardive dyskinetic movements over time. *Applied Nursing Research, 2*, 128–134.

E. Special Projects

1. Below is a list of five variables. Indicate briefly how you would operationalize each using structured observational procedures.
   a. Fear in hospitalized children
   b. Pain during childbirth
   c. Dependency in psychiatric patients
   d. Empathy in nursing students
   e. Cooperativeness in chemotherapy patients

2. Develop five problem statements for studies that could be implemented using observational procedures.

3. Develop a problem statement for a study that could be implemented using the participant–observer approach. Analyze the strengths and weaknesses of using this approach for your problem.

4. Suppose you wanted to study facial expressions in autistic children. Describe the sampling plan you would recommend for such a study.

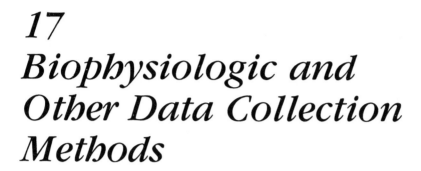

17
Biophysiologic and Other Data Collection Methods

A. Matching Exercises

Match each descriptive statement regarding a data collection approach from Set B with one (or more) of the statements from Set A. Indicate the letter(s) corresponding to your response next to each item in Set B.

SET A
a. Biophysiologic measure
b. Vignette
c. Projective technique
d. Q-sort
e. Delphi technique
f. None of the above

SET B	**RESPONSE**
1. Typically involves respondents' self-reports	_____
2. May require advanced training for interpretation	_____
3. Does not depend upon respondents' conscious cooperation to provide information about themselves	_____
4. Focuses on behaviors and events	_____

5. Is susceptible to response set biases   _____
6. Can be used to measure personality characteristics   _____
7. Can yield or involve qualitative data   _____
8. Involves a multiple iteration approach   _____
9. Yields ipsative data   _____
10. Can be administered by mail   _____

B. Completion Exercises

Write the words or phrases that correctly complete the sentences below.

1. Measures that are taken directly within a living organism are _____ _____ measures.
2. The entire set of apparatus and equipment used in connection with biophysiologic measurements is referred to as the _____ _____ .
3. A(n) _____ is a device that converts one form of energy into another.
4. A(n) _____ is a device for converting bioelectric potentials into electronic potentials.
5. The equipment used to amplify or modify an electronic signal is the _____ _____ equipment.
6. When biophysiologic materials are extracted from subjects and subjected to analysis, the data are referred to as _____ _____ measures.
7. The major advantage of using existing records is that it is _____ _____ .
8. In a Q-sort, subjects are generally instructed to place most of the cards near the _____ of the distribution.
9. In Q-sorts, forcing subjects to place a predetermined number of cards in each pile helps eliminate _____ _____ .
10. Because of its forced-choice nature, the Q-sort technique yields _____ _____ measures.

11. Respondents in a Delphi study are referred to as a(n) _____

_____ .

12. The Thematic Apperception Test (TAT) is an example of the _____

_____

method of projective techniques.

13. The projective technique in which subjects are presented with a verbal stimulus to

which to react is known as a(n) _____

_____ technique.

14. Critics of projective techniques claim that these methods are incapable of objec-

tive _____

_____ .

15. _____

are brief descriptions of persons or situations to which subjects are asked to react.

C. Study Questions

1. Define the following terms. Compare your definition with the definition in Chapter 17 of the textbook or in the glossary.

    a. Biophysiologic measure: _____

    _____

    _____

    b. Instrumentation system: _____

    _____

    _____

    c. Records: _____

    _____

    _____

    d. Selective deposit bias: _____

    _____

    _____

    e. Q-sort: _____

_____

_____

f. Normative measures: _____

_____

_____

g. Delphi technique: _____

_____

_____

h. Projective techniques: _____

_____

_____

i. Sentence-completion technique: _____

_____

_____

2. Below are five statements that might appear on Q-sort cards. For each, describe different continua according to which the cards could be sorted (e.g., one continuum could be "very much like me/not at all like me" for a statement such as "I like to go to parties.").

   a. Americans should be better edu-
     cated with respect to nutrition.   _____

   b. Nursing students need to under-
     stand the fundamentals of re-
     search methods.   _____

   c. Acid indigestion   _____

   d. Good fringe benefits   _____

   e. A course on human sexual devel-
     opment   _____

3. Indicate which of the measures below is an *in vivo* measure and which is an *in vitro* measure:

   a. Direct blood pressure measures   _____

   b. ECG measures   _____

   c. Hemoglobin concentration   _____

    d. Total lung capacity   _____

    e. Blood gas analysis of P_{CO_2} _____

    f. Chronoscope measures   _____

    g. Nasopharyngeal culture   _____

    h. Goniometer readings   _____

    i. Palmar Sweat Index   _____

    j. Blood pH   _____

4. Three nurses researchers were collaborating on a study of the effect of preoperative visits to surgical patients by operating room nurses on the stress levels of those patients just prior to surgery. One researcher wanted to use the patients' self-reports to measure stress; the second suggested using pulse rate and the Palmer Sweat Index; the third recommended using an observational measure of stress. Which measure do you feel would be the most appropriate for this research problem? Can you suggests other possible measures of stress that might be even more appropriate? Justify your response.

5. Suppose you were interested in studying nurses' reactions to working in an intensive care unit. Develop five incomplete sentences that could be used to obtain the information by the sentence-completion technique.

    a. _____

    b. _____

    c. _____

    d. _____

    e. _____

6. Identify five types of available records readily accessible to nurses that could be used to conduct a research study.

    a. _____

    b. _____

    c. _____

    d. _____

    e. _____

7. What are some of the advantages and disadvantages of a Q-sort, compared with a Likert scale?

ADVANTAGES   **DISADVANTAGES**

_____   _____

_____   _____

_____   _____

_____   _____

D. Application Exercises

Luhn (1991)* used a combination of projective techniques to study children's fears of hospitalization. Forty children were randomly assigned to an experimental or control condition. The experimental group received a special treatment designed to alleviate prehospitalization anxiety in school-age children. Controls did not receive any special instruction or treatment. The groups were then compared in terms of their responses to several projective measures, including the following:

- Responses to three cartoons that showed a hospitalized child interacting with hospital staff in three settings (as the child was being taken to the operating room; as the child was given medication; and as the child was eating). The children were asked to complete the dialogue by indicating the response of the hospitalized child.
- Sentence completions that included the following stems:
  I think nurses are. . .
  Being in a hospital is. . .
  I feel. . .
- Play technique involving the use of dolls. Two dolls are given to the child, and the child is asked to play out a scene between a hospitalized child and a playmate, who comes to visit him or her in the hospital.

1. Read and critique the description of Luhn's activities. Suggest possible alternative ways of collecting the data for the research problem. To assist you in your critique, here are some guiding questions:

   a. Which of the methods described in this chapter did the researcher employ? Was this a good selection? Would you recommend that the researcher switch to an alternative method, such as other methods described in Chapter 17, or in Chapters 14 through 16? Why or why not?

   *This example is fictitious.

 b. Comment on the technique(s) used in terms of response set biases.

 c. Comment on the technique(s) used in terms of the degree of objectivity of measuring the critical variables.

 d. Comment on the technique(s) used in terms of the efficiency of the procedure (i.e., amount of time required by subjects and researcher vis-à-vis the amount of data yielded).

 e. Comment on the technique(s) in terms of appropriateness for the study sample.

2. Below are several suggested research articles in which a projective technique was used. Review one of the articles and respond to questions a to e from Question D.1 above, to the extent possible, in terms of this actual study.

- Damrosch, S. (1985). Nursing students' assessments of behaviorally self-blaming rape victims. *Nursing Research, 34,* 221–224.
- George, T.B. (1982). Development of the self-concept of nurse in nursing students. *Research in Nursing and Health, 5,* 191–197.
- Wood, S.P. (1983). School-aged children's perceptions of the causes of illness. *Pediatric Nursing, 9,* 101–104.

Wilmot (1990)* conducted a quasi-experimental study of the effectiveness of a program for treating the physiologic anemia associated with pregnancy. The experimental treatment involved instruction regarding a nutritional regimen. The experimental group received verbal instructions by a nurse–midwife regarding dietary requirements and a list of foods known to be high in iron. Recommended daily amounts of certain foods were prescribed. The intervention also involved follow-up telephone conversations with the experimental group members at the 30th and 34th week of the pregnancy to discuss dietary and nutritional concerns. The comparison group members were given information that is normally given to pregnant women, with no individual follow-up. Fifty pregnant women who were outpatients at one hospital clinic served as the experimental subjects and 50 pregnant women who were clients at an HMO served as the comparison group subjects. Wilmot chose hematocrit readings as the measure of effectiveness of the experimental intervention. During the sixth month of the pregnancy, and again at the 36th-week visit, a hematocrit laboratory test was performed. The data were analyzed by comparing the degree of change that had occurred in the two hematocrit readings within the two groups. The researcher found that there were no significant differences in physiological anemia in the two groups, as measured by the changes in hematocrit tests.

3. Review and critique this study. Suggest alternative ways of collecting the data for the research problem. To assist you in your critique, here are some guiding questions:

  *This example is fictitious.

a. The data in this study were collected by a biophysiologic measure. Could the data have been collected in another way? In your opinion, should they have been?

b. Is the measure used an *in vivo* or *in vitro* type of measurement? Is it an invasive or noninvasive type of procedure?

c. Comment on the objectivity of the data collection method. How does its objectivity compare with other methods of measuring the dependent variable (e.g., observations of pallor of the skin, mucous membranes, and fingernail beds)?

d. What other biophysiologic measures might have been used to collect data in the study?

4. Below are several suggested research articles in which a biophysiologic method was used. Review one of the articles and respond to questions a to d from Question D.3 above, to the extent possible, in terms of this actual study.

- Doerring, L. and Dracup, K. (1988). Comparisons of cardiac output in supine and lateral positions. *Nursing Research*, *37*, 114–118.
- Levine-Silverman, S. and Johnson, J. (1990). Pulmonary artery pressure measurements. *Western Journal of Nursing Research*, *12*, 488–496.
- Stevenson, J.S. and Topp, R. (1990). Effects of moderate and low intensity long-term exercise by older adults. *Research in Nursing and Health*, *13*, 209–218.
- Wright, J. and Gong, H. (1990). "Auto-PEEP": Incidence, magnitude, and contributing factors. *Heart and Lung*, *19*, 352–357.

E. Special Projects

1. Develop a hypothesis in which each of the following could be used as measurements of the dependent variable:

a. ECG readings

b. Glucose concentration in the blood

c. Vital capacity

d. Body temperature

e. ACTH levels

f. Microbiological culture of sputum

g. Blood volume

h. Blood pressure

i. Red blood cell count

j. Reaction time

2. Suppose that you wanted to evaluate the effect of an experimental nursing intervention on the well-being and comfort of cardiac patients. Indicate several biophysiologic measures you might consider using in such a study. Evaluate each of your suggestions with respect to ease of obtaining the data, relevance, and objectivity.

3. Suppose that you were studying patients' opinions about the elements of care that are important to them during hospitalization. Develop 15 statements that might be used in a Q-sort for such a study. One example might be "Receive explanation about what is being done to me and why."

4. Using procedures described in Chapter 17, suggest ways of collecting data on the following: fear of death among the elderly; body image among amputees; reactions to the onset of menarche; anxiety; quality of life; nurses' morale in an emergency room; and dependence among cerebral palsied children.

18
Criteria for Assessing and Selecting Measuring Tools

A. *Matching Exercises*

Match each statement from Set B with one of the phrases from Set A. Indicate the letter corresponding to your response next to each of the statements in Set B.

SET A
a. Reliability
b. Validity
c. Both reliability and validity
d. Neither reliability nor validity

SET B   **RESPONSE**

1. Is concerned with the accuracy of measures.   _____

2. The measures must be high on this in order for the results of
   a study to be valid.   _____

3. If a measure possesses this, then it is necessarily valid.   _____

4. Can in some cases be estimated by procedures that yield a
   quantified coefficient.   _____

5. Can be enhanced by lengthening (adding subparts to) the
   measure.   _____

6. Is always improved when the measure is made more efficient.   _____

7. May in some cases be assessed by scrutinizing the components (subparts) of the measure. _____

8. Is necessarily high when the measure is high on objectivity. _____

9. Represents the proportion of true variability in a measure to total obtained variability. _____

10. Is concerned with whether the researcher has adequately conceptualized the variables under investigation. _____

B. Completion Exercises

Write the words or phrases that correctly complete the sentences below.

1. Obtained scores almost always consist of an error component and a _____ _____ component.

2. From a measurement perspective, response set biases represent a source of _____ .

3. A reliable measure is one that maximizes the _____ _____ component of observed scores.

4. Test–retest reliability focuses on the _____ _____ of a measure.

5. A _____ is an index of the strength and direction of a relationship between two variables.

6. When the values on one variable tend to be high among persons who score low on a second variable, the relationship is described as _____ .

7. Another term for internal consistency is _____ .

8. Procedures that examine the proportion of agreements between two independent judges yield estimates of _____ .

9. An instrument that is not reliable cannot be _____ .

10. The type of validity that focuses on the representativeness of the subparts of a measure is _____ validity.

11. The type of validity that deals with the ability of an instrument to distinguish individuals who differ in terms of some future criterion is _____ _____ validity.

12. _____ refers to evidence that different methods of measuring a concept yield comparable results.

13. _____ refers to evidence that a concept being measured is different from other similar concepts.

14. An instrument that makes good use of the time required to obtain measurements is described as _____ _____ .

15. An instrument that can make fine discriminations for different amounts of an attribute is described as high on _____ _____ .

C. Study Questions

1. Define the following terms. Compare your definition with the definition in Chapter 18 of the textbook or in the glossary.

   a. Obtained score: _____ _____ _____

   b. Error of measurement: _____ _____ _____

   c. Reliability: _____ _____ _____

   d. Test–retest reliability: _____ _____ _____

e. Reliability coefficient: _____

_____

_____

f. Internal consistency: _____

_____

_____

g. Split-half technique: _____

_____

_____

h. Spearman–Brown prophecy formula: _____

_____

_____

i. Cronbach's alpha: _____

_____

_____

j. Interrater reliability: _____

_____

_____

k. Validity: _____

_____

_____

l. Content validity: _____

_____

_____

m. Criterion-related validity: _____

_____

_____

n. Construct validity: _____

_____

_____

o. Known-groups technique: _____

_____

_____

p. Multitrait multimethod matrix: _____

_____

_____

q. Triangulation: _____

_____

_____

r. Psychometric assessment: _____

_____

_____

2. Use the Spearman–Brown prophecy formula to compute the following:
   a. The full reliability of a 12-item scale whose split-half reliability (i.e., based on six items) is .62.
   b. The approximate number of items that would have to be added to increase the reliability of a scale from .70 (for ten items) to .85.
   c. The decrease in reliability for a scale with 30 items and a reliability of .90 if five items were eliminated.

   a. _____

   b. _____

   c. _____

3. The reliability of measures of which of the following attributes would *not* be appropriately assessed using a test–retest procedure with one month between administrations. Why?
   a. Attitudes toward abortion: _____

   _____

   _____

   b. Stress: _____

   _____

   _____

    c. Achievement motivation: _____

    _____

    _____

    d. Nursing effectiveness: _____

    _____

    _____

    e. Depression: _____

    _____

    _____

4. Comment on the meaning and implications of the following statement:
A researcher found that the internal consistency of her 20-item scale measuring attitudes toward nurse–midwives was .74, using the Cronbach alpha formula.

    _____

    _____

    _____

    _____

    _____

5. In the following situation, what might some of the sources of measurement error be?
A sample of 100 nurses who worked in a large metropolitan hospital were asked to complete a 10-item Likert scale designed to measure job satisfaction. The questionnaires were distributed by nursing supervisors at the end of shifts. The staff nurses were asked to complete the forms and return them immediately to their supervisors.

    _____

    _____

    _____

    _____

    _____

6. Identify what is incorrect about the following statements:

   a. "My scale is highly reliable, so it must be valid."

   _____

   _____

   b. "My instrument yielded an internal consistency coefficient of .80, so it must be stable."

   _____

   _____

   c. "The validity coefficient between my scale and a criterion measure was .40; therefore, my scale must be of low validity."

   _____

   _____

   d. "My scale had a reliability coefficient of .80. Therefore, an obtained score of 20 is indicative of a true score of 16."

   _____

   _____

   e. "The validation study proved that my measure has construct validity."

   _____

   _____

   f. "My measure of stress was highly reliable in my study of primiparous women; you should use it in your study of stress among emergency room staff."

   _____

   _____

   g. "My advisor examined my new measure of dependence in nursing-home residents and, based on its content, assured me the measure was valid."

   _____

   _____

D. Application Exercises

Wait (1991)* wanted to study paternal bonding and attachment among men who had recently become fathers. Her main objective was to compare paternal attachment among men who had participated with their wives in prenatal classes and were present during childbirth with men who had not. In reviewing prior work in this area, Wait was unable to identify a paternal attachment scale that she found suitable to her needs. Therefore, she developed her own scale to measure paternal attachment. Her scale consisted of ten statements that respondents were asked to rate as "Very much like me," "Somewhat like me," or "Not at all like me." An example of the statements on the scale is "The birth of my baby aroused sentiments of immediate affection, closeness, and pride." Total scores were obtained by using procedures analagous to those used for summated rating scales. Wait pretested her scale with 30 men within 48 hours of the delivery of their babies. The internal consistency of the scale was assessed using the split-half technique, which, when corrected using the Spearman–Brown formula, yielded a reliability coefficient of .68. In terms of validating the instrument, Wait used two approaches. First, she invited two colleagues who worked in maternal–child nursing to review the ten statements and evaluate them in terms of content validity. Second, she asked nurses who worked in the hospital maternity ward to provide ratings, on a 0 to 10 scale, of how attached each new father appeared to be, based on the nurses' observations of the fathers' behavior vis-à-vis their babies. The correlations between the fathers' scale scores and the nurses' ratings was .56.

1. Review and critique this research effort. Suggest alternative ways of assessing the reliability and validity of the instrument. To assist you in your critique, here are some guiding questions:

   a. What method was used to assess the reliability of the instrument? On what aspect of reliability does this method focus? Is this focus appropriate? Should some alternative method for estimating reliability have been used? Should an *additional* method of estimating reliability have been used?

   b. Comment on the adequacy of the instrument's reliability. Should the reliability be better? If so, what might the researcher do to improve the reliability?

   c. What method was used to assess the validity of the instrument? On what aspect of validity does this approach focus? Is this focus appropriate? Should some alternative method for estimating validity have been used? Should an *additional* method of estimating validity have been used?

   d. Comment on the adequacy of the instrument's validity. Should the validity be better? If so, what might the researcher do to improve the validity?

*This example is fictitious.

    e. Comment on the efficiency, sensitivity, objectivity, and reactivity of the instrument.

2. Below are several suggested research articles. Read one of these articles, paying special attention to the ways the researcher assessed the adequacy of his or her measuring tool. Evaluate the measurement strategy, using questions a to e from Question D.1 as a guide. (Ignore the more technical aspects of the report, such as those that deal with factor analysis.)

- Frank-Stromberg, M. (1989). Reaction to the diagnosis of cancer questionnaire: Development and psychometric evaluation. *Nursing Research*, *38*, 364–369.
- Miller, J. F. and Powers, M. J. (1988). Development of an instrument to measure hope. *Nursing Research*, *37*, 6–9.
- Pollock, S. E. and Duffy, M. E. (1990). The Health-Related Hardiness Scale: Development and psychometric analysis. *Nursing Research*, *39*, 218–222.
- Thomas, S. D., Hathaway, D. K., and Arheart, K. L. (1990). Development of the General Health Motivation Scale. *Western Journal of Nursing Research*, *12*, 318–335.

E. Special Projects

1. Suppose that you were developing an instrument to measure attitudes toward "test-tube" babies. Your measure consists of 15 Likert-type items. Describe what you would do to: (a) estimate the reliability of your scale and (b) assess the validity of your scale.

2. Suggest the type of groups that might be used to validate measures of the following concepts using the known-groups technique:

    a. Self-esteem

    b. Empathy

    c. Capacity for self-care

    d. Emotional dependence

    e. Depression

    f. Hopelessness

    g. Health-promoting practices

    h. Health motivation

    i. Body image

    j. Coping capacity

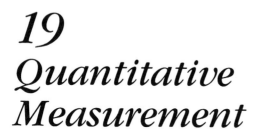

19
Quantitative Measurement

A. Matching Exercises

Match each variable in Set B with the level of measurement from Set A that captures the highest possible level for that variable. Indicate the letter corresponding to your response next to each variable in Set B.

SET A
a. Nominal scale
b. Ordinal scale
c. Interval scale
d. Ratio scale

SET B   **RESPONSE**

1. Hours spent in labor before childbirth   _____

2. Religious affiliation   _____

3. Reaction time   _____

4. Responses to Guttman scale items   _____

5. Temperature on the centigrade scale   _____

6. Nursing specialty area   _____

7. Status on the following scale: nonsmoker; light smoker; heavy smoker   _____

8. Pulse rate   _____

9. Score on a 25-item Likert scale   _____

10. Highest degree or certification attained   _____

11. Apgar scores   _____

12. Membership in ANA   _____

B. Completion Exercises

Write the words or phrases that correctly complete the sentences below.

1. People are not measured directly; their _____
_____ are measured.

2. The process of _____
refers to the assignment of numerical information to indicate how much of an attribute is present.

3. In measurement, numbers are assigned according to specified _____
_____ .

4. In order for a measure to be perfectly isomorphic to reality, the obtained scores must be identical to _____
_____ .

5. Nominal measurement involves a simple _____
_____ of objects according to some criterion.

6. Nominal-level data cannot be treated mathematically, but the data can be
_____ .

7. Rank-order questions are an example of _____
_____ measures.

8. With ratio-level measures there is a real, rational _____
_____ .

9. Unlike ordinal measures, interval measures involve _____
_____ between points on the scale.

10. Variables measured at one level can be converted to a _____
_____ level, but not vice versa.

C. Study Questions

1. Define the following terms. Compare your definition with the definition in Chapter 19 of the textbook or in the glossary.

   a. Measurement: _____

   _____

   _____

   b. Universe: _____

   _____

   _____

   c. Isomorphic: _____

   _____

   _____

   d. Nominal measurement: _____

   _____

   _____

   e. Ordinal measurement: _____

   _____

   _____

   f. Interval-level measurement: _____

   _____

   _____

   g. Ratio measurement: _____

   _____

   _____

2. For each of the following variables, specify the *highest* possible level of measurement that a researcher could attain.
   a. Attitudes toward the mentally handicapped   _____
   b. Birth order   _____
   c. Length of labor   _____

d. White blood cell count   _____

e. Marital status   _____

f. Tidal volume   _____
g. Scholastic Aptitude Test (SAT)
    scores   _____

h. Unit assignment for nursing staff   _____

i. Motivation for achievement   _____

j. Amount of sputum   _____

3. Name five biophysiologic measures that yield ratio-level measurements.

    a. _____

    b. _____

    c. _____

    d. _____

    e. _____

4. Name five biophysiologic measures that yield interval-level measurements.

    a. _____

    b. _____

    c. _____

    d. _____

    e. _____

5. Below are the salaries (fictitious) of ten hospital staff members. Convert these ratio-level measures to interval, ordinal, and nominal measures.

RATIO	INTERVAL	ORDINAL	NOMINAL
$ 8,500			
26,750			
53,000			
19,000			
18,500			
23,750			
29,000			
19,000			
28,750			
33,500			

D. Application Exercises

Fox (1991)* hypothesized that sleeping problems in infants were related to various conditions and experiences during childbirth. Fifty infants aged three to six months were diagnosed as having severe sleep-disturbance problems. A group of 50 infants aged three to six months who had normal sleeping patterns was used as the control group. Fox obtained the hospital records for all 100 children. The two groups were compared in terms of the following variables: amount of anesthesia administered during labor and delivery (none, small amount, large amount); length of time in labor (number of hours and minutes); type of delivery (cesarean or vaginal); birthweight (in grams); and Apgar scores at three minutes (score from one to ten). Fox found that the sleep-disturbance group had had significantly longer time in labor than the control group. The groups were comparable in terms of the other variables.

1. Review and critique this research effort. Suggest alternative measurement approaches. To assist you in your critique, here are some guiding questions:

   a. How many variables were measured in this study?

   b. For each variable, identify the level of measurement that was used.

   c. For each variable, indicate whether the measurement could have been made at a higher level of measurement than the level that was used. If yes, specify how you might measure the variable to obtain a higher level measure.

   d. For two of the variables, write out operational definitions that clearly indicate the rules of measurement for those variables.

2. Below are several suggested research articles. Skim one or more of these articles, paying special attention to the ways in which the research variables were operationalized. Evaluate the researcher's measurement strategy, using questions a to d from Exercise D.1 as a guide.

   • Boggs, P., Brown-Molnar, C.S., and DeLapp, T.D. (1988). Nurses' drug knowledge. *Western Journal of Nursing Research, 10,* 84–93.

   • Brown, B., Roberts, J., Browne, G., Byrne, C., Love, B., and Streiner, D. (1988). Gender differences in variables associated with psychosocial adjustment to a burn injury. *Research in Nursing and Health, 11,* 23–30.

   • Metzger, B.L. and Therrien, B. (1990). Effect of position on cardiovascular response during the Valsalva maneuver. *Nursing Research, 39,* 198–202.

   • Munroe, D.J. (1990). The influence of registered nurse staffing on the quality of nursing home care. *Research in Nursing and Health, 13,* 263–270.

---

*This example is fictitious.

- Weinbacher, F.M., Littlejohn, C.E., and Conley, P.F. (1990). Growth of bacteria in prefilled syringes stored in home refrigerators. *Applied Nursing Research, 3*, 63–67.

E. Special Project

Develop a problem statement (or a hypothesis) for a nursing research study. Prepare operational definitions that specify measurement rules for the variables in your statement. Identify for each variable the level of measurement your definition implies.

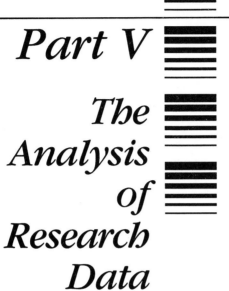

Part V

The Analysis of Research Data

20
Quantitative Analysis: Descriptive Statistics

A. Matching Exercises

Match each statement or phrase from Set B with one of the phrases from Set A. Indicate the letter corresponding to your response next to each of the statements in Set B.

SET A
a. Measure(s) of central tendency
b. Measure(s) of variability
c. Measure(s) of neither central tendency nor variability
d. Measure(s) of both central tendency and variability

SET B	**RESPONSE**
1. The range	_____
2. In lay terms, an average	_____
3. A percentage	_____
4. A parameter	_____
5. Descriptor(s) of a distribution of scores	_____
6. Descriptor(s) of how heterogeneous a set of values is	_____
7. A standard deviation	_____
8. The mode	_____
9. Can be plotted on histograms	_____
10. Coincide in a normal distribution	_____

B. Completion Exercises

Write the words or phrases that correctly complete the sentences below.

1. A descriptive index (e.g., percentage) from a sample is called a(n) _____

   _____ .

2. Researchers using quantitative analysis apply _____

   _____

   to draw conclusions about a population based on information from a sample.

3. A(n) _____
   is a systematic arrangement of quantitative data from lowest to highest values.

4. In the equation $\sum f = n$, the n represents the total _____

   _____ .

5. Histograms and _____
   are the two most common ways of presenting frequency information in graphic
   form.

6. A distribution is described as _____
   if the two halves are mirror images of each other.

7. A distribution is _____
   skewed if its longer tail points to the left.

8. A distribution that has only one peak is said to be _____

   _____ .

9. Many human characteristics such as height and intelligence are distributed to

   approximate a(n) _____

   _____ .

10. Measures that summarize the "typical" value in a distribution are known as mea-

    sures of _____

    _____ .

11. The symbol $\overline{X}$ is usually used by researchers to designate the _____

    _____ .

12. In a positively skewed distribution, the index indicating the "average" value that
    would be the farthest of the three indices to the left would be the _____

    _____ .

13. Measures of _____
are concerned with how spread out the data are.

14. When scores are not very spread out (dispersed over a wide range of values), the sample is said to be _____

_____ with respect to that variable.

15. The _____
indicates one half of the range of scores within which the middle 50% of the scores lie.

16. The difference between an individual raw score and the mean is known as a

_____ .

17. A squared standard deviation is referred to as a _____

_____ .

18. Statistics for two variables examined simultaneously are called _____

_____ .

19. Another term for a contingency table is a(n) _____

_____ .

20. A graphic representation of a correlation between two variables is referred to as

a(n) _____

_____ .

21. Relationships are described as _____

_____

if high values on one variable are associated with low values on a second.

22. The most commonly used correlation index is _____

_____ .

C. Study Questions

1. Define the following terms. Compare your definition with the definition in Chapter 20 of the textbook or in the glossary.

   a. Parameter: _____

b. Histogram: _____

_____

_____

c. Skewed distribution: _____

_____

_____

d. Bimodal distribution: _____

_____

_____

e. Normal curve: _____

_____

_____

f. Mode: _____

_____

_____

g. Median: _____

_____

_____

h. Mean: _____

_____

_____

i. Range: _____

_____

_____

j. Standard deviation: _____

_____

_____

k. Contingency table: _____

_____

_____

l. Correlation: _____

_____

_____

2. Prepare a frequency distribution and histogram for the following set of scores, which represent the ages of 30 women receiving estrogen replacement therapy:

47 50 51 50 48 51 50 51 49 51
54 49 49 53 51 52 51 52 50 53
49 51 52 51 50 55 48 54 53 52

Describe the resulting distribution in terms of its symmetry and modality.

3. Calculate the mean, median, and mode for the following pulse rates:

78 84 69 98 102 72 87 75 79 84 88 84 83 71 73

Mean: _____

Median: _____

Mode: _____

4. At the top of page 168 is a contingency table from an SPSS[x] printout. The table presents data from a study of sexually active teenagers in which both males and females were asked how old they were when they first learned about birth control. Each row in the table indicates the ages specified by the respondents. The last row contains the code for respondents who could not remember how old they were, coded "88." Answer the following questions about this contingency table:

a. How many males were included in the study?

b. How many females learned about birth control at age 14?

c. What percentage of respondents were 16 when they learned about birth control?

d. What percentage of males did not know at what age they learned about birth control?

e. Of those respondents who were 13 when they learned about birth control, what percentage was female?

```
SPSS BATCH SYSTEM

FILE   NONAME   (CREATION DATE = 08/18/90)

* * * * * * * * * * * * * * * *  C R O S S T A B U L A T I O N
    V276        HOW OLD WHEN FIRST LEARNED BC              BY SEX
* * * * * * * * * * * * * * * * * * * * * * * * * * * * * * * *

                          SEX
                 COUNT  I
                 ROW PCT IMALE,      FEMALE      ROW
                 COL PCT I                       TOTAL
                 TOT PCT I      1.I       2.I
    V276         --------I--------I--------I
                 13.  I.    13  I     10  I      23
                      I   56.5  I   43.5  I    13.9
                      I   15.7  I   12.0  I
                      I    7.8  I    6.0  I
                     -I--------I--------I
                 14.  I    14  I     16  I      30
                      I   46.7  I   53.3  I    18.1
                      I   16.9  I   19.3  I
                      I    8.4  I    9.6  I
                     -I--------I--------I
                 15.  I     7  I     14  I      21
                      I   33.3  I   66.7  I    12.7
                      I    8.4  I   16.9  I
                      I    4.2  I    8.4  I
                     -I--------I--------I
                 16.  I     8  I      2  I      10
                      I   80.0  I   20.0  I     6.0
                      I    9.6  I    2.4  I
                      I    4.8  I    1.2  I
                     -I--------I--------I
                 17.  I     1  I      1  I       2
                      I   50.0  I   50.0  I     1.2
                      I    1.2  I    1.2  I
                      I    0.6  I    0.6  I
                     -I--------I--------I
                 88.  I     3  I      2  I       5
                      I   60.0  I   40.0  I     3.0
                      I    3.6  I    2.4  I
                      I    1.8  I    1.2  I
                     -I--------I--------I
                 COLUMN      83         83        166
                 TOTAL     50.0       50.0      100.0
```

5. Write out the meaning of each of the following symbols:

a. Σ _____

b. $\overline{X}$ _____

c. f _____

d. n _____

e. X _____

f. x _____

g. SD _____

h. δ^2 _____

D. Application Exercises

Hudson (1991)* hypothesized that patients with a high degree of physical mobility would perceive themselves as being healthier than patients with less physical mobility. To test this hypothesis, 120 male patients in a VA hospital were asked to rate themselves on a five-point scale regarding their current physical health (1 = very unhealthy and 5 = very healthy) and to predict the number of days that they would be hospitalized. Forty of these patients had been categorized as "of limited mobility," another 40 were classified as "of moderate mobility," and the remaining 40 were described as "of high mobility." Hudson reported a portion of his findings as follows:

> The self-ratings of physical health were fairly normally distributed for the sample as a whole: 42% rated themselves as neither healthy nor unhealthy; 7% and 21% described themselves as "very healthy" or "somewhat healthy," respectively. At the other extreme, 6% said they were "very unhealthy" and 24% said "somewhat unhealthy." The three groups differed in their ratings, however. In the high-mobility group, a full 45% said they were either "very" or "somewhat healthy," while only 30% of the moderate-mobility and 15% of the low-mobility groups said this. For the entire sample, the mean predicted length of stay was 14.1 days. The median length, however, was only 12.5 days. For the three groups, the means and standard deviations with respect to predicted length of stay in hospital were as follows:
>
> | | MEAN | STANDARD DEVIATION |
> |---|---|---|
> | High Mobility | 7.1 | 3.2 |
> | Moderate Mobility | 11.9 | 4.5 |
> | Low Mobility | 23.3 | 7.4 |
>
> In this sample of patients, the correlation between predicted length of stay in hospital and the health rating was .56.

1. Review and critique this study, particularly with respect to the statistical analysis. To assist you in this critique, here are some guiding questions:

   a. Was the mode of data analysis (i.e., quantitative versus qualitative) appropriate? Why or why not?

   b. Which of the following types of statistical analysis were used in this example?

      Frequency distribution
      Measure of central tendency
      Measure of variability
      Contingency table
      Correlation

*This example is fictitious.

    c. Comment on the appropriateness of each statistic reported in the example. Is the statistic appropriate given the level of measurement of the variable? Does the statistic throw away information? Is the statistic the most stable statistic possible?

    d. Identify two or three statistics that were not reported by the researcher that could have been reported given the data that were collected. Evaluate the extent to which the absence of this information weakened (or streamlined) the report of the results.

    e. Discuss the meaning of the means and standard deviations reported in this example.

2. Below are several suggested research articles. Skim one (or more) of these articles and respond to questions a to e from Exercise D.1 in terms of the actual research study. (At this point, ignore the references to tests of statistical significance, which are covered in the next chapter.)

- Andrews, C. M. and Chrzanowski, M. (1990). Maternal position, labor, and comfort. *Applied Nursing Research, 3,* 7–13.
- Hogan, N. S. and Balk, D. E. (1990). Adolescent reactions to sibling death: Perceptions of mothers, fathers, and teenagers. *Nursing Research, 39,* 103–106.
- Kearney, M. H., Cronenwett, L. R. and Barrett, J. A. (1990). Breast-feeding problems in the first week postpartum. *Nursing Research, 39,* 90–95.
- Primomo, J., Yates, B. C., and Woods, N. F. (1990). Social support for women with chronic illness. *Research in Nursing and Health, 13,* 153–161.
- Tulman, L. and Fawcett, J. (1988). Return of functional ability after childbirth. *Nursing Research, 37,* 77–81.

E. Special Projects

1. Fictitious data from 24 nurses for six variables are presented on the facing page. Compute and present five to ten different statistics that you think would best summarize this information.

SUBJECT NO.	SHIFT[a]	ANXIETY SCORES[b]	SUPERVISOR'S PERFORMANCE RATING[c]	NO. OF YEARS OF EXPERIENCE	MARITAL STATUS[d]	JOB SATISFACTION SCORE[e]
1	1	10	4	5	2	4
2	1	13	4	2	2	5
3	1	8	2	1	1	3
4	1	4	7	10	1	3
5	1	6	9	12	1	4
6	1	9	8	7	1	2
7	1	12	6	8	2	4
8	1	5	4	2	1	5
9	2	10	5	4	2	1
10	2	14	6	1	2	4
11	2	8	5	3	1	5
12	2	15	8	2	2	2
13	2	11	8	7	2	3
14	2	14	7	9	1	1
15	2	1	5	3	2	2
16	2	8	8	6	1	3
17	3	3	7	19	2	4
18	3	7	4	7	1	1
19	3	19	5	1	2	2
20	3	5	6	11	1	1
21	3	8	3	2	1	3
22	3	10	4	5	2	2
23	3	13	6	6	2	1
24	3	14	5	3	1	2

[a]1 = day; 2 = evening; 3 = night
[b]Scores are from a low of 0 to a high of 20, 20 = most anxious
[c]Ratings are from 1 = poor to 9 = excellent
[d]1 = married; 2 = not married
[e]Scores are from low of 1 to high of 5; 5 = most satisfied

2. Ask 25 friends, classmates, or colleagues the following four questions:

- How many brothers and sister do you have?
- How many children do you expect to have in total?
- Would you describe your family during your childhood as "close," or "not very close"?
- On your 14th birthday, were you living with both biological parents, one biological parent, or with neither biological parent?

When you have gathered your data, calculate and present several statistics that describe the information you obtained.

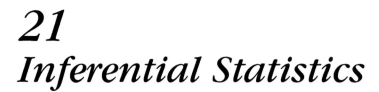

21
Inferential Statistics

A. *Matching Exercises*

Match each phrase or statement from Set B with one of the phrases in Set A. Indicate the letter corresponding to your response next to each of the statements in Set B.

SET A
a. Parametric test(s)
b. Nonparametric test(s)
c. Neither parametric nor nonparametric tests
d. Both parametric and nonparametric tests

SET B	**RESPONSE**
1. The signed rank test	_____
2. Paired *t*-test	_____
3. Researcher establishes the risk of Type I errors	_____
4. Used when a score distribution is nonnormal	_____
5. Offers proof that the null hypothesis is either true or false	_____
6. Assumes the dependent variable is measured on an interval or ratio scale	_____
7. Uses sample data to estimate population values	_____
8. Kruskal–Wallis test	_____
9. Computed statistics are compared to tabled values based on theoretical distributions	_____
10. Yields confidence intervals	_____

11. Used most frequently by nurse researchers   _____
12. Used to compare differences for three groups   _____
13. ANOVA   _____
14. Pearson's *r*   _____
15. Chi-square test   _____

B. Completion Exercises

Write the words or phrases that correctly complete the sentences below.

1. Sampling distributions of means have a _____ _____ distribution.

2. The standard error of the mean is estimated by dividing the sample SD by the square root of the _____ _____ .

3. The Greek letter mu (μ) usually symbolizes the _____ _____ .

4. The degree of risk of making a _____ _____ error is controlled by the researcher.

5. Tests that involve the estimation of parameters are referred to as _____ _____ tests.

6. The term *distribution-free statistics* is sometimes applied to_____ _____ tests.

7. The most commonly used _____ _____ are the .05 and .01 levels.

8. Using a .01 rather than a .05 level increases the risk of committing a _____ _____ error.

9. The _____ test is used to compare two groups on the basis of deviations from the median.

10. The statistic computed in an analysis of variance is the _____ _____ statistic.

11. In an analysis of variance, the term analogous to the *variance* is referred to as the _____ .

12. Multifactor ANOVA permits a test of differential effects of one variable for all levels of a second variable, or a test of the _____ _____ hypothesis.

13. The nonparametric test analogous to ANOVA is called the _____ _____ test.

14. In chi-square analyses, observed frequencies are compared to _____ _____ .

15. Spearman's rho is a nonparametric analog of _____ _____ .

16. When both the independent and dependent variables are nominal measures, the most commonly used test statistic is the _____ _____ .

17. Kendall's tau is used when both the independent and dependent variables are _____ measures.

18. Pearson rs among a set of variables, when presented in a two-dimensional format, yield a _____ _____ .

19. The _____ is an index describing the magnitude of relationship between two dichotomous variables.

20. If a research report stated that a statistical test yielded a $p > .05$, the result would generally be considered _____ _____ .

C. Study Questions

1. Define the following terms. Compare your definition with the definition in Chapter 21 of the textbook or in the glossary.

   a. Sampling error: _____
   _____
   _____

b. Sampling distribution: _____

_____

_____

c. Standard error of the mean: _____

_____

_____

d. Point estimation: _____

_____

_____

e. Confidence interval: _____

_____

_____

f. Null hypothesis: _____

_____

_____

g. Type I error: _____

_____

_____

h. Type II error: _____

_____

_____

i. Level of significance: _____

_____

_____

j. Statistical significance: _____

_____

_____

k. Nonparametric tests: _____

_____

l. Degrees of freedom: _____

_____

_____

m. *t*-test: _____

_____

_____

n. Analysis of variance: _____

_____

_____

o. Multiple comparison procedures: _____

_____

_____

p. Chi-square test: _____

_____

_____

2. A nurse researcher measured the amount of time (in minutes) spent in recreational activities by a sample of 200 hospitalized paraplegics. She compared male and female patients, as well as those aged 50 and younger versus those over 50. The four group means were as follows:

	MALE	**FEMALE**
≤ 50	98.2 ($N = 50$)	70.1 ($N = 50$)
> 50	50.8 ($N = 50$)	68.3 ($N = 50$)

A two-way ANOVA yielded the following results:

	F	**df**
Sex	3.61	1,196
Age group	5.87	1,196
Sex × Age group	6.96	1,196

Determine the levels of significance of these results and interpret their meaning.

3. The correlation between the number of days absent per year and annual salary in a sample of 100 employees of an insurance company was found to be −.23. Discuss this result in terms of significance levels and meaning.

4. Indicate which statistical test(s) you would use to analyze data for the following variables:
   a. Variable 1 is psychiatric patients' sex; Variable 2 is whether or not the patient has attempted suicide in the past 12 months.

   _____

   _____

   b. Variable 1 is the participation versus nonparticipation of patients with a pulmonary embolus in a special treatment group; Variable 2 is the pH of the patients' arterial blood gases.

   _____

   _____

   c. Variable 1 is serum creatinine concentration levels; Variable 2 is daily urine output.

   _____

   _____

   d. Variable 1 is patients' marital status (married versus not married); Variable 2 is the patients' degrees of self-reported depression (mild versus moderate versus severe).

   _____

   _____

5. Below is a correlation matrix produced by an SPSS^x run. The variables in this matrix are as follows:

   CMATURE = career maturity test scores
   EMPKNOW = employment knowledge test scores
   BCKNOW = birth control knowledge test scores
   V326 = attitudes toward working mothers
   FAMSIZE = number of siblings

   Answer the following questions with respect to this matrix:
   a. How many respondents completed the Career Maturity test?
   b. What is the correlation between employment knowledge and birth control knowledge?
   c. Is the correlation between family size and career maturity significant at conventional levels?
   d. What is the level of significance between employment knowledge and attitudes toward working mothers?
   e. With which variable(s) is career maturity significantly related at conventional levels?
   f. Explain what is meant by the correlation between CMATURE and BCKNOW.

```
SPSS BATCH SYSTEM                                     FRI, NOV 20, 1990,  8:48 AM

FILE   NONAME    (CREATION DATE = 11/20/90)
SUBFILE   REDIR1

- - - - - - - - - - - P E A R S O N    C O R R E L A T I O N    C O E F F I C I E N T S - - - - -


           CMATURE     EMPKNOW     BCKNOW      V326       FAMSIZE

CMATURE    1.0000       .4618       .3309       .0057      -.0136
           (  334)     (  330)     (  333)     (  175)     (  324)
           S=#####     S= .000     S= .000     S= .470     S= .404

EMPKNOW     .4618      1.0000       .2725       .1502      -.0639
           (  330)     (  333)     (  332)     (  174)     (  323)
           S= .000     S=#####     S= .000     S= .024     S= .126

BCKNOW      .3309       .2725      1.0000      -.0129      -.0830
           (  333)     (  332)     (  338)     (  177)     (  328)
           S= .000     S= .000     S=#####     S= .432     S= .067

V326        .0057       .1502      -.0129      1.0000      -.0947
           (  175)     (  174)     (  177)     (  178)     (  175)
           S= .470     S= .024     S= .432     S=#####     S= .106

FAMSIZE    -.0136      -.0639      -.0830      -.0947      1.0000
           (  324)     (  323)     (  328)     (  175)     (  329)
           S= .404     S= .126     S= .067     S= .106     S=#####
```

(COEFFICIENT/(CASES)/SIGNIFICANCE) (A VALUE OF 99.0000 IS PRINTED IF A COEFFICIENT CANNOT BE COMPUTED)

D. Application Exercises

Cummings (1991)* investigated whether taste acuity declines with age, using a cross-sectional design. Eighty subjects were given a taste acuity test in which they were asked to indicate, for 25 substances, whether the taste was salty, sweet, bitter, or sour. The substances were presented in randomized order. Each person had five scores: four scores corresponding to the correct identification of the substances in the four taste categories, and one total score. Twenty subjects from each of the following age groups were tested: 31–40; 41–50; 51–60; and 61–70. It was hypothesized that taste acuity would decline with age, both overall and for all four subcategories of taste. The mean test scores for the four groups on all five outcome measures are presented below, together with information on the statistical tests performed.

	AGE GROUP						
	31–40	*41–50*	*51–60*	*61–70*	*F*	*df*	*p*
Salty Test	6.3	5.8	5.7	5.4	3.5	3,76	<.05
Sweet Test	5.0	5.0	5.4	5.2	1.2	3,76	>.05
Bitter Test	4.0	4.1	3.7	3.3	2.6	3,76	<.05
Sour Test	1.9	2.0	2.0	2.1	0.8	3,76	>.05
Overall Test	17.2	16.9	16.8	16.0	2.4	3,76	<.05

*This example is fictitious.

Cummings concluded that her hypothesis was only partially supported by the data.

1. Review and critique the above study. Suggest possible alternatives for handling the analysis of the data. To assist you in your critique, here are some guiding questions:

   a. For each of the variables, indicate the actual level of measurement as used; now indicate the highest possible level of measurement for each. Is there a discrepancy? If so, can you think of a justification for it?

   b. What statistical test was used to analyze the data? Did the researcher use the appropriate statistical test? If not, what statistical test do you think would be more suitable?

   c. Are the degrees of freedom as presented correct?

   d. The test statistics shown are associated with a specified p level. Using the tables in the Appendix of the textbook, determine whether these p levels are correct.

   e. Which of the results is statistically significant? Describe the meaning of each of the statistical tests.

2. Below are several suggested research articles. Skim one (or more) of these articles and respond to questions a to e from Exercise D.1 in terms of the actual research study.

   • Miller, K. M. and Perry, P. A. (1990). Relaxation technique and postoperative pain in patients undergoing cardiac surgery. *Heart and Lung, 19*, 136–146.
   • Murata, J. M. (1990). Father's family violence and son's delinquency. *Western Journal of Nursing Research, 12*, 60–74.
   • Rice, V. H., Sieggreen, M., Mullin, M., and Williams, J. (1988). Development and testing of an arteriography information intervention for stress reduction. *Heart and Lung, 17*, 23–27.
   • Schmieding, N. J. (1990). A model for assessing nurse administrators' actions. *Western Journal of Nursing Research, 12*, 293–306.
   • Smith, L. S. (1988). Ethnic differences in knowledge of sexually transmitted diseases in North American black and Mexican American migrant farmworkers. *Research in Nursing and Health, 11*, 51–58.

E. Special Projects

1. Below is a list of variables. Assume that you have data from 500 nurses on these variables. Develop two or three hypotheses regarding the relationships among these variables and indicate what statistical tests you would use to test your hypotheses.

- Number of years of nursing experience
- Type of employment setting (hospital, nursing school, public school system, etc.)
- Salary
- Marital status
- Job satisfaction ("dissatisfied," "neither dissatisfied nor satisfied," or "satisfied")
- Number of children under age 18
- Sex
- Type of nursing preparation (diploma, Associate's, Bachelor's)

2. Using the data presented in Exercise E.1 of Chapter 20, perform at least two inferential statistical tests. Write a one-paragraph description of the results.

22

Advanced Statistical Procedures

A. Matching Exercises

Match each phrase from Set B with one (or more) of the statistical analyses presented in Set A. Indicate the letter corresponding to your response next to each of the statements in Set B.

SET A
a. Multiple regression analysis
b. Discriminant function analysis
c. Factor analysis
d. Canonical correlation
e. Multivariate ANOVA

SET B   **RESPONSE**

 1. Always has more than one independent variable   _____
 2. Is based on least-squares principles   _____
 3. Yields an R^2 statistic   _____
 4. Used to reduce variables to a smaller number of dimensions _____
 5. Has more than one dependent variable   _____
 6. Yields a Wilk's lambda statistic   _____
 7. Is a multivariate statistical procedure   _____
 8. May use a procedure known as principal components   _____
 9. Involves a dependent variable that is categorical (nominal) _____
10. Can involve as few as three variables   _____

B. Completion Exercises

Write the words or phrases that correctly complete the sentences below.

1. In the basic linear regression equation $(Y = a + bX)$, b is referred to as the

   _____ .

2. In a regression context, the error terms are referred to as _____

   _____ .

3. The square of _____ indicates the proportion of variance accounted for by two or more correlated variables.

4. The _____ coefficient is never less than the highest bivariate correlation between the independent or dependent variables.

5. Independent variables are introduced one at a time in _____

   _____ multiple regression.

6. Scores that have been adjusted to have a mean of zero and a standard deviation of one are called _____ .

7. Standardized regression coefficients are referred to as _____

   _____ .

8. ANCOVA is shorthand for _____

   _____ .

9. In ANCOVA, the extraneous variable being controlled is referred to as the

   _____ .

10. _____

    is the procedure that yields mean scores adjusted for covariates.

11. In factor analysis, the underlying dimensions are referred to as _____

    _____ .

12. The first phase in factor analysis is the _____

    _____ phase.

13. In factor analysis, _____

    _____ are values equal to the sum of the squared weights for each factor.

14. The second phase of factor analysis is the _____

    _____ phase.

15. In _____

    rotation, factors are kept at right angles to one another, while in _____

    _____

    rotation the factors are allowed to be correlated.

16. The procedure known as _____
    can be used for classification purposes.

17. The most general multivariate procedure is _____

    _____ .

18. MANOVA is the acronym for _____

    _____ .

19. In path analysis, the conceptual causal model is depicted in a _____

    _____ .

20. A variable whose determinants lie outside of a model in path analysis is called

    _____ .

21. When a causal flow is unidirectional, the model is said to be _____

    _____ .

22. In power analysis, the four major factors needed to arrive at a solution are the

    significance criterion, the power criterion, the sample size, and the _____

    _____ .

C. Study Questions

1. Define the following terms. Compare your definition with the definition in Chapter 22 of the textbook or in the glossary.

   a. Multivariate statistics: _____

      _____

      _____

   b. Multiple regression analysis: _____

      _____

      _____

c. Least-squares principle: _____

_____

_____

d. Coefficient of determination: _____

_____

_____

e. Analysis of covariance: _____

_____

_____

f. Factor analysis: _____

_____

_____

g. Factor loadings: _____

_____

_____

h. Factor scores: _____

_____

_____

i. Discriminant function analysis: _____

_____

_____

j. Canonical correlation: _____

_____

_____

k. Multivariate analysis of variance: _____

_____

_____

l. Path analysis: _____

_____

_____

m. Mediating variable: _____

_____

_____

n. Power analysis: _____

_____

_____

o. Eta-squared: _____

_____

_____

p. Life table analysis: _____

_____

_____

q. LISREL: _____

_____

2. Examine the correlation matrix below and explain the various entries. Explain why the *multiple* correlation coefficient between Variables B through E and Satisfaction with Parenthood is .54. Could it be smaller? How could it be made larger? What is the R^2 for this set of variables? What does this mean?

	VAR. A	VAR. B	VAR. C	VAR. D	VAR. E
	Satisfaction With Parenthood	Number of Children	Marital Status (Married vs. Divorced/ Widowed)	Family Income	Religion (Catholic vs. Non-Catholic)
Var. A	1.00				
Var. B	− .26	1.00			
Var. C	.48	.29	1.00		
Var. D	.19	− .22	.68	1.00	
Var. E	.10	.37	.17	− .04	1.00

3. Suggest possible covariates that could be used in the following analyses:
   a. An analysis of the effect of family stress on the incidence of child abuse:

_____

_____

b. An analysis of the effect of age on patients' acceptance of pastoral counseling:

_____

_____

c. An analysis of the effect of therapeutic touch on patients' perceptions of well-being: _____

_____

_____

d. An analysis of the effect of need for achievement on students' attrition from a nursing program: _____

_____

_____

e. An analysis of the effect of faculty rank on faculty members' satisfaction with communications among colleagues: _____

_____

_____

4. In the following examples, which multivariate procedure is most appropriate for analyzing the data?
   a. A researcher is testing the effect of verbal expressiveness, self-esteem, age, and the availability of family supports among a group of recently discharged psychiatric patients on recidivism (i.e., whether they will be readmitted within 12 months after discharge).

   _____

   _____

   b. A researcher is comparing the bereavement and coping processes of recently widowed versus divorced individuals, controlling for their age and length of marriage.

   _____

   _____

   c. A researcher wants to test the effects of (a) two drug treatments and (b) two dosages of each drug on (a) blood pressure and (b) the pH and PO_2 levels of arterial blood gases.

   _____

   _____

d. A researcher wants to predict hospital staff absentee rates based on month of the year, staff rank, shift, number of years with the hospital, and marital status.

_____

_____

5. Below is a list of variables that a nurse researcher might be interested in predicting. For each, suggest at least three independent variables that could be used in a multiple regression analysis.
   a. Leadership in nursing supervisors:

   _____

   _____

   b. Nurses' frequency of administering pain medication:

   _____

   _____

   c. Proficiency in doing patient interviews:

   _____

   _____

   d. Patient satisfaction with nursing care:

   _____

   _____

   e. Anxiety levels of prostatectomy patients:

   _____

   _____

D. Application Exercises

Wolpin (1991)* studied psychological distress and life satisfaction in a sample of 100 infertile/sterile couples. She hypothesized that the individuals' psychological reactions would differ depending on whether the fertility problem was their own or that of their partners. She further hypothesized that women would be more negatively affected psychologically than men by the fertility problem. Wolpin administered anonymous questionnaires to both husbands and wives who were patients at an infertility clinic. In 50 couples, the fertility problem was

*This example is fictitious.

diagnosed as a male problem, and in the remaining 50 couples it was diagnosed as a female problem. The questionnaire included a set of 50 items, designed to measure psychological well-being. The items included such statements as "I have felt moments of severe depression lately" and "My husband (wife) and I have been less communicative than usual." Respondents were asked to indicate whether each statement was "very much like me," "somewhat like me," or "not at all like me." Responses to the 50 items were then factor analyzed. Four factors were extracted and rotated orthogonally. Wolpin labelled the four factors as follows: "Depression," "Marital Satisfaction," "Optimisim about the Future," and "Feelings of Sex-Role Inadequacies." The factor scores on these four scales were analyzed in four separate (2 × 2) analyses of covariance, using the women's age and duration of the marriage as covariates. The following table summarizes the results of the statistical tests for the main and interaction effects (for each test there are 1 and 194 degrees of freedom):

	SEX OF PARTNER	LOCUS OF FERTILITY PROBLEMS	SEX × LOCUS INTERACTION
	(Male versus female)	*(Self versus partner)*	
Depression	F = 5.9* $p < .05$	F = 6.7† $p < .01$	F = 3.9 $p < .05$
Marital Satisfaction	F = 0.8 ns	F = 1.4 $p < .05$	F = 2.3 ns
Optimism	F = 1.9 ns	F = 2.1 ns	F = 1.5 ns
Sex-Role Inadequacy	F = 5.2* $p < .05$	F = 11.4† $p < .001$	F = 3.1 ns

*Wife higher than husband
†Self higher than partner
ns = not statistically significant

Wolpin concluded that her hypotheses were partially supported by the data.

1. Review and critique this study with respect to the analysis of the data. To assist you in your critique, here are some guiding questions:

   a. For each variable in the study, what is the level of measurement?

   b. How many independent and dependent variables are there in this study?

   c. Considering responses to the above two questions and the size of the sample, did the researcher use the appropriate analysis? Suggest alternative ways to analyze the data and compare the information yielded in the two approaches.

   d. The test statistics shown are associated with a specific p level. Using the tables in the Appendix of the text, determine whether each p level is correct.

   e. What does each of the statistical tests signify?

2. Below are several suggested research articles. Read one of these articles, paying special attention to the analysis of the data. Respond to questions a to e from Exercise D.1. in terms of the actual research study.

   • Herth, K. (1990). Relationship of hope, coping styles, concurrent losses, and setting to grief resolution in the elderly widow(er). *Research in Nursing and Health, 13,* 109–117.

- Kearney, M., Cronenwett, L. R. and Barrett, J. A. (1990). Breast-feeding problems in the first week postpartum. *Nursing Research, 39,* 90–95.
- Littlefield, V. M., Chang, A., and Adams, B. N. (1990). Participation in alternative care. *Research in Nursing and Health, 13,* 17–25.
- Mattson, S. (1990). Coping and developmental maturity of R.N. Baccalaureate students. *Western Journal of Nursing Research, 12,* 514–524.
- Nickel, J. T., Brown, K. J., and Smith, B. A. (1990). Depression and anxiety among chronically ill heart patients. *Research in Nursing and Health, 13,* 87–97.

E. Special Projects

1. On the following page is a rotated factor matrix for a set of 20 Likert items administered to 300 teenagers in a study of teenage sexuality and contraceptive practices.

   Using this matrix, do the following:

   a. Identify and label the underlying dimensions.
   b. Select the items that will form three scales.
   c. Compute factor scores for three individuals whose responses to the 20 items are as follows:

Mary:	1	2	5	3	5	4	2	3	4	4
	3	1	1	4	2	1	4	1	2	4
Tom:	4	1	2	4	1	2	5	4	1	3
	1	2	4	2	1	3	4	5	2	3
Debbie:	2	4	1	2	2	1	5	1	2	4
	4	5	2	2	5	1	1	4	5	4

2. Design and describe a study in which you would use both factor analysis and discriminant function analysis.

3. Design and describe a study in which you would use life table analysis.

ITEM	FACTOR I	FACTOR II	FACTOR III
1. It is primarily the woman's responsibility to use birth control.	.10	.62	.22
2. It is difficult to talk to your boyfriend about what kind of birth control the two of you should use.	.09	-.07	.36
3. It can be exciting to take a chance on getting pregnant.	.72	-.03	.08
4. It is relatively easy to put the worry about pregnancy out of one's mind.	.18	-.02	.25
5. It is sometimes important to prove your love by taking a chance.	.48	-.21	.13
6. No form of birth control really works.	.18	.06	-.18
7. People are foolish to depend on luck when it comes to pregnancy risk.	-.40	.17	-.23
8. Every teen who really wants to use birth control can easily do so.	.16	-.02	-.47
9. Sometimes making love with a particular person is worth the chance of pregnancy.	.51	.11	-.12
10. The best birth control methods are those that the man uses.	-.09	-.42	.17
11. A woman sometimes has a really hard time avoiding sexual involvement even when there isn't any birth control available.	.05	-.04	.32
12. The problem with some birth control is that you have to plan for the possibility of intercourse ahead of time.	-.04	.03	.52
13. A woman can't really trust a man to handle contraception.	-.01	.39	.07
14. If you really love someone, the chances of pregnancy aren't so important.	.36	.12	-.01
15. Getting hold of good birth control is a lot of effort and bother.	.02	-.09	.61
16. A woman needs to be in control of birth control for her own protection.	.03	.43	-.15
17. It's pretty easy to protect oneself against a pregnancy.	-.11	.06	-.68
18. Having unprotected sex isn't worth the risk of disrupting your life.	-.58	-.07	.24
19. It's really a hassle to use birth control.	.22	-.01	.49
20. It's a man's duty to see that his partner is protected.	.08	-.47	-.20

23
The Analysis
of Qualitative Data

A. Matching Exercises

Match each descriptive statement from Set B with one (or more) of the statements from Set A. Indicate the letter corresponding to your response next to each item in Set B.

SET A
a. Analytic induction approach
b. Grounded theory approach
c. Content analysis
d. None of the above

SET B   RESPONSE

1. Can be facilitated through use of computers   _____
2. Involves the technique known as constant comparison   _____
3. Typically involves quantification   _____
4. Involves the development of an inductively derived hypothesis   _____
5. Involves the analysis of narrative materials   _____
6. Requires data saturation   _____
7. Can use an experimental design   _____
8. Requires data to be categorized and coded   _____

9. Can be used to collect psychological data   _____

10. Alternates between tentative explanation and definition   _____

B. Completion Exercises

Write the words or phrases that correctly complete the sentences below.

1. The term *holistic* is more often used to describe _____

_____ than

_____ research.

2. In qualitative research, hypothesis _____

_____ is frequently a goal.

3. The main task in organizing qualitative data involves the development of a(n)

_____ .

4. In developing a conceptual file, the researcher must devise a comprehensive

_____ .

5. The analysis of qualitative data generally begins with a search for _____

_____ .

6. The use of _____

involves an accounting of the frequency with which certain themes and relationships are supported by the data.

7. The approach known as _____

involves an interactive process in which qualitative data are used to pose questions and arrive at tentative explanations.

8. The approach known as _____

involves a constant comparative approach to collecting and analyzing qualitative data, with an eye toward theory development.

9. In content analysis, the unit of analysis referred to as the _____

_____

signifies an entire message or production.

10. If the unit of analysis in a content analysis were words, whole pages of a large

document might be selected as the _____

_____ .

C. *Study Questions*

1. Define the following terms. Compare your definition with the definition in Chapter 23 of the textbook or in the glossary.

    a. Qualitative analysis: _____

    _____

    _____

    b. Administrative files: _____

    _____

    _____

    c. Analytic files: _____

    _____

    _____

    d. Quasi-statistics: _____

    _____

    _____

    e. Grounded theory: _____

    _____

    _____

    f. Content analysis: _____

    _____

    _____

    g. Constant comparison: _____

    _____

    _____

    h. Flow chart: _____

    _____

    _____

    i. Space-and-time measure: _____

    _____

2. For each of the problem statements below, indicate whether you think a re-searcher should collect primarily qualitative or quantitative data. Justify your response.

a. How do victims of AIDS cope with the discovery of their illness?

_____

_____

_____

b. What important dimensions of nursing practice differ in developed and underdeveloped countries?

_____

_____

_____

c. What is the effect of therapeutic touch on patient well-being?

_____

_____

_____

d. Do nurse practitioners and physicians differ in the performance of triage functions?

_____

_____

_____

e. Is a patient's length of stay in hospital related to the quality or quantity of his/her social supports?

_____

_____

_____

f. How does the typical American feel about such new reproductive tech-nologies as *in vitro* fertilization?

_____

_____

_____

g. By what processes do women make decisions about having an amniocentesis?

_____

_____

h. What are the psychological sequelae of having an organ transplant?

_____

_____

_____

i. What factors are most predictive of a woman giving birth to a very low birthweight infant?

_____

_____

_____

j. What effects does caffeine have on gastrointestinal motility?

_____

_____

_____

3. Read the excerpt below, taken from a real interview. Use the coding scheme in Table 23.1 of the text to code the topics discussed in this excerpt.

I think raising the children is so much easier without the father around. There isn't two people conflicting back and forth. You know, like . . . like you discipline them during the day. They do something wrong, you're not saying, "When daddy gets home, you're going to get a spanking." You know, you do that. The kid gets a spanking right then and there. But when two people live together, they have their ways of raising and you have your ways of raising the children and it's so hard for two people to raise children. It's so much easier for one person. The only reason a male would be around is financial-wise. But me and the kids are happier now, and we get along with each other better, cause like, there isn't this competitive thing. My husband always wanted all the attention around here.

D. Application Exercises

Logan (1990)* studied the phenomenon of "being on precautions" from the perspective of hospitalized adults. She began her study, after securing permission, by spending two days on the hospital units where the data would be

*This example is fictitious.

collected. The two days were spent familiarizing herself with the units, learning how best to collect the data, determining where she could position herself in an unobtrusive manner, and establishing a trusting relationship with the nursing staff.

The data for the study were collected using the techniques of observation and unstructured interviewing. Logan selectively sampled all times of the day and all days of the week in two-hour segments to make her observations. The time schedule began on a Monday morning at 7 AM and continued until 9 AM. On Tuesday, the observation time became 9 AM until 11 AM. Observations continued around the clock on consecutive days until no new information was being collected. Logan positioned herself either directly outside the door to the patient's room or sat in the patient's room to make her observations. Observations included any activity or interaction between the patient and hospital staff or between the patient and herself.

The unstructured interviewing process consisted of asking patients to clarify why they were doing certain things and what they liked or disliked about the hospital experience.

Logan recorded the observations and data from the interviews in a log immediately following each two-hour observation segment. All data were recorded in chronologic order. In addition to the above, Logan also recorded any feelings she had during the observation experience. As time progressed, she reread her field notes after every four hours of observation. As commonalities began to emerge from the data, she developed another section to her log according to similarity of content and referenced the daily log notes according to commonalities. Logan continued making observations until she felt she had a "feel for the data" and additional observations or interactions provided only redundant information. A total of five patients were observed.

Categories that emerged from the data were labeled "avoidance," "devaluation as a person," and "loneliness." Evidence for the avoidance perspective came from patient comments during informal conversations with the researcher and the observational field notes. The evidence included statements such as "Nurses seldom come into the room because they have to put all that [pointing to precaution gowns] stuff on"; "Look, she [the cleaning woman] won't come in the room. She's afraid of me"; "Did you see that? Only my doctor would touch me. The rest were afraid to touch me." Observational field notes contained several notations of nurses coming to the door of the room asking, "Do you want anything?" but not entering the room.

The category "devaluation as a person" emerged from comments such as "I don't like being treated as a specimen"; "Do you have to wear gloves every time you take care of me [made to a nurse]?"; "If I go to the door of the room, they [the nurses] yell at me [made to the researcher]."

The category "loneliness" was developed from field notes that observed patients occasionally putting the call light on to find out what time it was or how long until lunch, or asking about a noise they had heard. Comments that conveyed the same feeling of loneliness were "Being confined in this room is like being in jail"; "I can't wait to get out of here and have dinner with my friends"; and "The hours seem endless here."

1. Review and critique this study. Suggest alternative ways of collecting and analyzing the data for the research problem. To assist you in your critique, here are some guiding questions:

    a. Comment on the choice of research approach. Was a qualitative research approach suitable for the phenomenon being studied? In your opinion, would a more quantitative research approach have been more appropriate?

    b. The data in the study were collected by observation and informal interviewing. Could the data have been collected in another way? Should they have been?

    c. What type of sampling plan was used to sample observations in the study? Would an alternative sampling plan have been better? Why or why not?

    d. The researcher recorded her observations, feelings, and interviews immediately following each two-hour observation period. Comment on the appropriateness of this method. Can you identify any biases that could be present in this choice of method? Suggest alternative ways of recording the data.

    e. Categorize the field notes made in the study according to their purpose. What additional types of field notes would you have included?

    f. How did the researcher handle the concept of theoretical saturation? Could you recommend any improvements?

    g. What types of validation procedures did the researcher use? Can you suggest additional procedures that might have improved the study?

    h. Comment on the categories that emerged from the data. Do they seem to reflect accurately the data that were collected? Would you have developed different ones?

2. Below are several suggested research articles. Skim one or more of these articles and respond to questions a to h from Exercise D.1, to the extent possible, in terms of the actual research study.

    - Blenner, J. L. (1990). Attaining self-care in infertility treatment. *Applied Nursing Research, 3,* 98–104.

    - Jezewski, M. A. (1990). Culture brokering in migrant farmworker health care. *Western Journal of Nursing Research, 12,* 497–513.

    - Norberg, A. and Asplund, K. (1990). Caregivers' experience of caring for severely demented patients. *Western Journal of Nursing Research, 12,* 75–84.

    - VanDongen, C. J. (1990). Agonizing questioning: Experiences of survivors of suicide victims. *Nursing Research, 39,* 224–229.

E. Special Projects

1. Get ten or so people to write one or two paragraphs on their feelings about death and dying. Perform a thematic analysis of these paragraphs.

2. Develop two or three research questions that you think might lend themselves to a qualitative study.

3. Read one of the studies listed in the Suggested Readings of Chapter 23. Generate several hypotheses that could be tested based on the reported findings.

24
Integration of Qualitative and Quantitative Analysis

A. Matching Exercises

Match each descriptive statement from Set B with one of the statements from Set A. Indicate the letter corresponding to your response next to each item in Set B.

SET A
a. Qualitative data
b. Quantitative data
c. Both qualitative and quantitative data
d. Neither qualitative nor quantitative data

SET B	**RESPONSE**
1. Should be collected to help improve nursing practice	_____
2. Are especially useful for understanding dynamic processes	_____
3. Are often collected in large-scale surveys	_____
4. Are useful in proving the validity of theories	_____
5. Are usually collected by phenomenological researchers	_____
6. Can profit from triangulation	_____
7. Are often used in tests of causal relationships	_____
8. Can contribute to theoretical insights	_____
9. Require validity checks	_____
10. Tend to be collected from small samples	_____

B. Completion Exercises

Write the words or phrases that correctly complete the sentences below.

1. Qualitative and quantitative data are often _____

   _____
   in that they "mutually supply each other's lack."

2. The major conceptual frameworks of nursing demand neither _____

   _____ nor _____ data.

3. Progress in a developing area of research tends to be _____

   _____
   and can profit from multiple feedback loops.

4. A major advantage of integrating different approaches is potential enhancements

   to the study's _____

   _____ .

5. A frequent application of integration is in the development of research _____

   _____ .

6. In a quantitative study, the inclusion of qualitative data might facilitate the _____

   _____
   of the findings, and vice versa.

7. When qualitative data collection is embedded in a survey effort, it is often more

   productive to use a _____

   _____ approach.

8. In studies of the effects of complex interventions, qualitative data may be useful in

   addressing the _____

   _____ question.

9. A major barrier to integration is _____

   _____ biases.

10. Although an integrated data collection/analysis approach is _____

   _____ ,
   it can be argued that the collection of multiple types of data in a single study is
   efficient.

C. Study Questions

1. Define the following terms. Compare your definition with the definition in Chapter 24 of the textbook or in the glossary.

   a. Multimethod research: _____

   _____

   _____

   b. "Black box": _____

   _____

   _____

   c. Epistemological bias: _____

   _____

   _____

   d. Complementarity: _____

   _____

   _____

2. Read one of the following studies, in which qualitative data were gathered and analyzed to address a research question. Suggest ways in which the collection of quantitative data might have enriched the study, strengthened its validity, and/or enhanced its interpretability:

   - Blenner, J. L. (1990). Attaining self-care in infertility treatment. *Applied Nursing Research, 3,* 98–104.
   - DeVito, A. (1990). Dyspnea during hospitalization for acute phase of illness as recalled by patients with chronic obstructive pulmonary disease. *Heart and Lung, 19,* 186–191.
   - Tapp, R. A. (1990). Inhibitors and facilitators to documentation of nursing practice. *Western Journal of Nursing Research, 12,* 229–240.
   - VanDongen, C. J. (1990). Agonizing questioning: Experiences of survivors of suicide victims. *Nursing Research, 39,* 224–229.

3. Read one of the following studies, in which quantitative data were gathered and analyzed to address a research question. Suggest ways in which the collection of qualitative data might have enriched the study, strengthened its validity, and/or enhanced its interpretability:

   - Froman, R. D. and Owen, S. V. (1990). Mothers' and nurses' perceptions of infant care skills. *Research in Nursing and Health, 13,* 247–253.

- Halm, M. A. (1990). Effects of support groups on anxiety of family members during critical illness. *Heart and Lung, 19*, 62–71.
- Lindgren, C. L. (1990). Burnout and social support in family caregivers. *Western Journal of Nursing Research, 12*, 469–487.
- Schmieding, N. J. (1990). A model for assessing nurse administrators' actions. *Western Journal of Nursing Research, 12*, 293–306.

D. Application Exercises

Depner (1991)* conducted a study to investigate breastfeeding practices among teenage mothers, who have been found in many studies to be less likely than older mothers to breastfeed. Using birth records from two large hospitals, Depner contacted 250 young women between the ages of 15 and 19 who had given birth in the previous year and invited them to participate in a survey. Those who agreed to participate ($N = 185$) were interviewed by telephone (when possible), using a structured interview that asked about breastfeeding practices, attitudes toward motherhood, availability of social supports, and conflicting demands, such as school attendance or employment. Several psychologic scales (including measures of depression and self-esteem) were also administered. Teenagers without a telephone were interviewed in person in their own home. All of the teenagers interviewed at home were also interviewed in greater depth, using a topic guide that focused on such areas as feelings about breastfeeding, the decision-making process that led them to decide whether or not to breastfeed, barriers to breastfeeding, and intentions to breastfeed with any subsequent children. Depner used the quantitative data to determine the characteristics associated with breastfeeding status and duration. The qualitative data were used to interpret and validate the quantitative findings.

1. Review and critique this study. Suggest alternative data collection and analysis approaches. To assist you in your critique, here are some guiding questions:

   a. Which of the aims of integration, if any, were served by this study?

   b. What was the researcher's basic strategy for integration? How effective was this strategy in addressing the aims of integration?

   c. Suggest ways of altering the design of the study and the data collection approach to further promote integrative aims.

   d. Would the study have been stronger if it had involved the collection of quantitative data only? Qualitative data only? Why or why not?

---

*This example is fictitious.

2. Below are several suggested research articles of studies that used an integrated approach. Read one or more of these articles and respond to questions a to d from Exercise D.1 in terms of these actual research studies.

- Laffrey, S. L. and Pollock, S. E. (1990). An exploration of adult health behaviors. *Western Journal of Nursing Research*, *12*, 434–445.
- Pridham, K. F. Chang, A. S. and Hansen, M. (1987). Mothers' problem-solving skill and use of help with infant-related issues. *Research in Nursing and Health*, *10*, 263–275.
- Sohier, R. (1988). Multiple triangulation and contemporary nursing research. *Western Journal of Nursing Research*, *10*, 732–742.

E. Special Projects

1. Prepare five problem statements that would be amenable to multimethod research.

2. For one of the problems suggested in Exercise E.1, write a 2-3 page description of how the data would be collected, and how the use of both qualitative and quantitative data/analysis would strengthen the study.

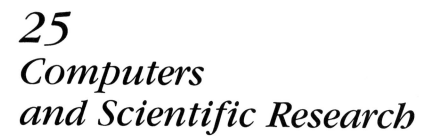

25
Computers
and Scientific Research

A. Matching Exercises

Match each statement from Set B with one of the terms in Set A. Indicate the letter corresponding to your response next to each of the statements in Set B.

SET A
a. Computer hardware
b. Computer software
c. Neither hardware nor software
d. Both hardware and software

SET B   RESPONSE

 1. Includes the central processing unit   _____
 2. Facilitates the analysis of research data   _____
 3. Is read into the computer via input devices   _____
 4. Makes use of programming languages   _____
 5. Is the part of the computer that does the thinking _____
 6. Includes magnetic tape drives   _____
 7. SPSS^x is one example   _____
 8. Requires electronics expertise to design this _____
 9. Includes the data collected by a researcher   _____
10. Can be used only in the interactive mode   _____

B. *Completion Exercises*

Write the words or phrases that correctly complete the sentences below.

1. The most distinctive characteristic of computers is their _____

   _____ .

2. I/O stands for _____

   _____ .

3. Data are read in through some form of _____

   _____ .

4. CPU stands for _____

   _____ .

5. The computer _____
   is composed of a series of cells, each of which stores an instruction or numerical
   value.

6. A set of instructions to the computer is referred to as a(n) _____

   _____ .

7. FORTRAN and BASIC are examples of _____

   _____ .

8. Magnetic tapes and magnetic disks are types of _____

   _____
   storage devices for a mainframe computer.

9. Line printers and plotters are examples of _____

   _____ .

10. Computer users can communicate directly with the computer via the _____

    _____ mode.

11. SPSS, SAS, and BMD-P are examples of _____

    _____ .

12. For security reasons, legitimate users of computer facilities often need a _____

    _____ .

C. Study Questions

1. Define the following terms. Compare your definition with the definition in Chapter 25 of the textbook or in the glossary.

   a. Computer hardware: _____

   _____

   _____

   b. Output device: _____

   _____

   _____

   c. Control unit: _____

   _____

   _____

   d. Arithmetic/logic unit: _____

   _____

   _____

   e. Computer software: _____

   _____

   _____

   f. Programming language: _____

   _____

   _____

   g. Compiler: _____

   _____

   _____

   h. Printout: _____

   _____

   _____

   i. Batch processing: _____

   _____

   _____

j. Turnaround time: _____

_____

_____

k. Time-sharing: _____

_____

_____

l. Mainframe computer: _____

_____

_____

m. Microcomputer: _____

_____

_____

n. Supercomputer: _____

_____

_____

o. BASIC: _____

_____

_____

p. BMD-P: _____

_____

_____

q. Byte: _____

_____

_____

r. Log on: _____

_____

_____

2. Examine Figure 25.3 in the textbook. Describe in your own words the flow of operations for processing the data and commands from the 30 subjects described in the "Available Programs" section. Indicate specific I/O devices that might be used.

3. In the example of the BASIC program presented in Chapter 25, suppose that instead of the average, you wanted to know the total sum. What change to the program would you need to make to obtain this information?

D. Application Exercises

Tienda,* a student researcher, was learning to prepare SPSS^x instructions to analyze her data. The data consisted of information for the following variables: subject's age, smoking status (smoker/nonsmoker), and number of days absent from work during 1990. A total of 125 men and women provided data for this study. Below are the SPSS^x instructions that Tienda initially prepared to obtain basic descriptive statistics such as frequency counts (e.g., number of smokers in her sample):

```
DATA LIST
        /1 AGE 1 SMOKESTATUS 2 DAYSABSNT 3
FREQUENCIES = AGE, SMOKESTATUS, DAYSABSNT
        /STATISTICS = ALL
BEGIN DATA
```

There are five errors in this set of instructions. Make the necessary changes to remove the errors.

E. Special Projects

1. Visit a computer center and ask for a tour of the mainframe hardware facilities. Make a list of the I/O devices available to users. Make a list of the statistical software packages available. Determine whether the facility operates in the batch mode, the interactive mode, or both.

2. As indicated throughout the text, research primarily focuses on the relationships between variables. For instance, in the example presented in the Application Exercise, above, the researcher would probably be interested in learning if the

*This example is fictitious.

average number of days absent is higher among smokers than nonsmokers. The SPSS^x command for this computation is as follows:

MEANS TABLES = VARX BY VARY

where VARX is the continuous dependent variable (here, number of days absent) and VARY is the categorical independent variable (smoking status).

Suppose that you were interested in studying birth outcomes in various groups of women. Suppose further that you have collected data from 150 women who have just given birth, with respect to the following variables: age group (under 20/20 and over); birthweight of infant (in ounces); Apgar score (from one to ten); ethnicity of mother (white/black/Hispanic); and type of delivery (vaginal/cesarean). Write out SPSS^x instructions that would (a) produce frequency information for these five variables; (b) compare the birthweights in the two age groups; and (c) compare the Apgar scores for the two types of delivery.

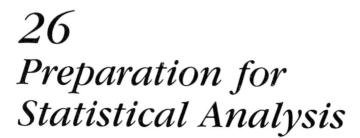

26
Preparation for Statistical Analysis

A. Matching Exercises

Match each variable listed in Set B with a field-width specification listed in Set A. Indicate the letter corresponding to your response (i.e., for the maximum field-width needed) next to each of the statements in Set B.

SET A
a. 1-digit field-width
b. 2-digit field-width
c. 3-digit field-width
d. 4-digit field-width
e. 5-digit field-width or wider

SET B   **RESPONSE**

1. Infant's birthweight (in ounces)   _____

2. Nurse's annual salary (in dollars)   _____

3. Number of beds in Hospital X   _____

4. Response to a Likert-type item   _____

5. Pulse rate   _____

6. Marital status   _____

7. Number of hours in surgery   _____

8. Tidal volume   _____

9. Weekly aspirin consumption   _____
10. Height in inches   _____
11. Number of cigarettes smoked per week   _____
12. Number of pregnancies   _____
13. Systolic blood pressure   _____
14. Student enrollment in a school of nursing   _____
15. Religion   _____

B. Completion Exercises

Write the words or phrases that correctly complete the sentences below.

1. Coding should ideally involve _____

   _____ symbols.

2. Variables measured on the _____

   _____ scale can be assigned an arbitrary code.

3. Variables that are inherently _____

   _____ do not need to be coded.

4. Closed-ended questions can usually be _____

   _____ .

5. In coding open-ended or unstructured materials, the coding categories should be

   mutually exclusive and _____

   _____ .

6. "Don't knows" and refusals must be treated as _____

   _____ .

7. Each individual case (e.g., each respondent) in a study should be assigned a

   unique _____

   _____ .

8. _____

   procedures are recommended to detect errors in data entry.

9. Entered data are not ready for analysis until they have been _____

   _____ .

10. Coding and data entry decisions should be fully _____ _____ .

11. Raw data often need to be _____ _____ or altered before proceeding to statistical analysis.

12. Two ways of handling the problem of missing data include (1) deletion of missing _____ and (2) deletion of the _____ .

C. Study Questions

1. Define the following terms. Compare your definition with the definition in Chapter 28 of the textbook or in the glossary.

   a. Coding: _____
   _____
   _____

   b. Intercoder reliability: _____
   _____
   _____

   c. Missing data: _____
   _____
   _____

   d. Fixed format: _____
   _____
   _____

   e. Free format: _____
   _____
   _____

f. Right-justification: _____

_____

_____

g. Field: _____

_____

_____

h. Edge-coding: _____

_____

_____

i. Outlier: _____

_____

_____

j. Consistency check: _____

_____

_____

k. Codebook: _____

_____

_____

l. Recoded data: _____

_____

_____

m. Ceiling effect: _____

_____

_____

n. Item reversal: _____

_____

_____

2. Respond to the questions posed in Figure 26. 1 of the textbook. Code your own responses and transfer them to a coding sheet. (If none is available commercially, construct your own, modeled on the coding sheet in Figure 26. 2.)

3. Complete the codebook that is started in Figure 26.3 (based on questions 5–11 of Figure 26.1).

4. Write out the SPSS instructions to create a composite variable called "ATTITUDE," based on the questions shown in Table 15.1 of the textbook. Remember to reverse the negatively worded questions.

5. Write out the SPSS instructions to create dichotomous variables for ANXIETY and SUPRATNG (Anxiety scores and Supervisor's performance ratings) for the data presented in Exercise E.1 in Chapter 20 in this Study Guide. Use the median of these two variables (which you will need to compute) to dichotomize the variables.

D. Application Exercises

Wise*, a student researcher, developed a preliminary coding layout for her questionnaire (which focused on the postgraduation experiences of nursing school students). A portion of that layout is presented on the following page, together with Wise's plans for coding missing data.

1. Review and critique the coding layout on the next page. Suggest improvements that you feel are needed. To assist you in your critique, here are some guiding questions:

   a. What is the maximum number of respondents that the coding scheme allows for?

   b. Check the field-width for each question. Are extra columns needed in order to code all possible responses? Are there too many columns allocated for some questions?

   c. Examine the coding categories specified for the precoded questions. Are they reasonable and consistent? Do they permit all responses to be adequately coded?

   d. Examine the missing data codes and comment on their appropriateness. Does the researcher distinguish between different types of missing data? If not, should she have? Do any of the missing codes conflict with actual codes? Recommend changes as necessary.

   *This example is fictitious. The example was not intended to reflect proper sequencing or distribution of questionnaire items, but was designed to include points covered in the text related to coding.

e. When you have made all the changes you believe are needed (if any), how many columns in total will be required in order to include all of the data produced for these ten questions?

TO BE ENTERED IN COLUMNS	MISSING VALUES CODE	QUESTION
1–4		ID Number

5	9	1. Are you currently employed?
		  1. yes
		  2. no (SKIP TO Q 7)

6	9	2. How many hours to you work in a typical week?_____
7–10	9	3. What is your monthly salary? $_____

11	9	4. In what type of setting are you currently employed?
		  1. hospital or clinic
		  2. nursing home
		  3. school
		  4. private practice
		  5. community agency
		  6. health-maintenance organization
		  7. industry
		  8. other: nursing-related settings
		  9. other: non-nursing-related settings

12–13	9	5. How many other nurses are employed by the same agency/institution that employs you?_____

14	9	6. How satisfied are you with your present position?
		  1. very satisfied
		  2. somewhat satisfied
		  3. neither satisfied nor dissatisfied
		  4. somewhat dissatisfied
		  5. very dissatisifed
		(SKIP TO Q9)

15	9	7. Are you currently seeking employment?
		  1. yes
		  2. no (SKIP TO Q 9)

16	9	8. Which of the following have you done in trying to find a job?
		  1. read newspaper ads
		  2. contacted my school's placement office
		  3. gone to an employment agency
		  4. called or written to institutions directly
		  5. called employed friends to see if they knew of any openings

17–18	9	9. How old are you?_____

19	9	10. What is your marital status?
		  1. single, never married
		  2. married
		  3. separated or divorced
		  4. widowed

E. Special Projects

1. Ask 10 to 15 of your friends to respond to the following question:

   What is the *one* least satisfying aspect about being a nurse, in your opinion?

   Develop codes for this question based on the themes expressed in the responses you obtain. Compare your coding scheme with that prepared by other fellow students.

2. Find a computer installation and ask a user assistant to instruct you in the use of a terminal. Respond to the questions from the Exercise D.1, and enter your data in the appropriate columns.

Part VI

Communication in the Research Process

27
Interpreting and Reporting Research Results

A. Matching Exercises

Match each sentence from Set B with one of the sections in a research report in which these sentences would appear, as listed in Set A. Indicate the letter corresponding to your response next to each of the statements in Set B.

SET A
a. Introduction
b. Methods section
c. Results section
d. Discussion section

SET B   **RESPONSE**

1. The sample consisted of 50 men aged 65 to 75, selected at
   random from a nursing home.   _____

2. These data suggest that nurses have become increasingly less
   accepting of traditional sex-role stereotypes.   _____

3. It is hypothesized that male and female paraplegics differ in
   their perceptions of the importance of architectural barriers.   _____

4. The 100 subjects were randomly assigned to the experimental
   and control groups using a random-numbers table.   _____

5. Mothers who breastfed their babies were significantly more likely than those who did not to express favorable views toward the motherhood role ($t = 3.2$, $df = 98$, $p < .01$). _____

6. A major flaw of these early studies was the low reliability of the instruments the researchers used. _____

7. The findings reported here are consistent with the work of Hogan (1990) and Crimmins (1988), both of whom used as subjects patients with MI. _____

8. Age at marriage was found to be significantly related to both educational attainment ($r = -.25$) and number of children ($r = -.38$). _____

B. Completion Exercises

Write the words or phrases that correctly complete the sentences below.

1. The first step in the interpretation of research findings involves an analysis of the

_____

of the results, based on various types of evidence.

2. It is useful for a researcher to perform a _____ when the results of the main hypothesis tests were not statistically significant.

3. In quantitative analysis, the results are generally in the form of

_____ and _____ .

4. Interpretation of results is easiest when the results are consistent with the researcher's _____ .

5. Since researchers are not generally interested in discovering relationships exclusively for the research sample, an important part of the interpretive process

involves an assessment of the _____ of the results.

6. An important research precept is that _____

_____

does not prove causation.

7. Nonsignificant findings mean that the null hypothesis is _____ ;

significant findings mean that the null hypothesis is _____ .

8. The _____
   section of a report discusses the researcher's aims, the research questions, and the context of the study.

9. The _____
   section of a report describes what the researcher did to gather and analyze the data.

10. Research findings are described in the _____
    _____ section of a report.

11. Statistical information can most effectively and succinctly be displayed in _____
    _____ .

12. Graphic presentations of statistical information are usually referred to as _____
    _____ .

13. Interpretations of results are normally presented in the _____
    _____

    section of a report.

14. The main communication outlet for scholarly research activity is _____
    _____ .

15. When a research report is authored by more than one person who made equal contributions, the names are listed _____ .

C. Study Questions

1. Define the following terms. Compare your definition with the definition in Chapter 27 of the textbook or in the glossary.

   a. Negative results: _____
   _____
   _____

   b. Positive results: _____
   _____
   _____

c. Mixed results: _____

_____

_____

d. Research report: _____

_____

_____

e. Summary: _____

_____

_____

f. Journal article: _____

_____

_____

g. "Blind" review: _____

_____

_____

h. Call for papers: _____

_____

_____

i. Poster session: _____

_____

_____

j. Refereed journal: _____

_____

_____

2. The following sentences all have stylistic flaws. Suggest ways in which the sentences could be improved.

ORIGINAL	IMPROVEMENT
a. ICU nurses experience more stress than nurses on a general ward ($t = 2.5$, $df = 148$, $p < .05$)	
b. "A Study Investigating the Effect of Primary Care Nursing on the Emotional Well-Being of Patients in a Cardiac Care Unit."	
c. The nonsignificant results demonstrate that there is no relationship between diet and hyperkinesis.	
d. It has, therefore, been proven that people have a more negative body image if the age of onset of obesity is before age 20.	
e. The positive significant relationship indicates that occupational stress causes sleep disturbances.	

3. Below are several suggested research articles in which the researchers obtained mixed results—that is, some hypotheses were supported and others were not. Review and critique the researcher(s) interpretation of the findings for one or more of these studies and suggest some possible alternatives.

   - Engle, V. (1986). The relationship of movement and time to older adults' functional health. *Research in Nursing and Health*, 9, 123–129.
   - Mickschl, D. B., Davidson, L. J., Flournoy, D. J., and Parker, D. E. (1990). Contamination of enteral feedings and diarrhea in patients in intensive care units. *Heart and Lung*, 19, 362–370.
   - Miller, K. M. and Perry, P. A. (1990). Relaxation technique and postoperative pain in patients undergoing cardiac surgery. *Heart and Lung*, 19, 136–146.
   - Naylor, M. D. (1990). Comprehensive discharge planning for hospitalized elderly: A pilot study. *Nursing Research*, 39, 156–161.
   - White, M. A. *et al.* (1990). Sleep onset latency and distress in hospitalized children. *Nursing Research*, 39, 134–139.

4. Read the research report by Gretchen Randolph entitled "Therapeutic and physical touch: Physiological response to stressful stimuli," which appeared in the

January 1984 issue of *Nursing Research* (Volume 33, pages 33–36). None of the researcher's hypotheses were supported. Review and critique Randolph's interpretation of the findings for one or more of these studies and suggest some possible alternatives.

5. Suppose that you were the author of a research article with the titles indicated below. For each, name two different journals to which your article could be submitted for publication.
   a. "Parental attachment to children with Down's syndrome."

   _____

   _____

   b. "Sexual functioning among men in their 70s."

   _____

   _____

   c. "Comparison of therapists' and clients' expectations regarding psychiatric therapy."

   _____

   _____

   d. "The effects of fetal monitoring on selected birth outcomes."

   _____

   _____   _____

   e. "Effectiveness of alternative methods of relieving pressure sores."

   _____

   _____

6. Suggest titles for five of the studies described in the "Application" sections of this workbook.

D. Application Exercises

Olsen (1990)* hypothesized that preschool children from single-parent families are more likely than those from two-parent families to display negative behavioral and psychosocial patterns. She administered a behavioral checklist to 30

*This example is fictitious.

divorced mothers and 30 married mothers who accompanied their preschool child (age 3–5) during immunization for measles. Each mother was asked to indicate the frequency with which these preschool children exhibited a series of behaviors ("very often," "fairly often," "sometimes," or "never"). Examples of the behavioral items include "Often cries with little or no apparent reason," "Tends to sulk when unable to have his or her own way," and "Has trouble making or keeping friends." The items were combined to form three subscales: Home and Family; Friends and Peers; and General. A total "Behavioral Adjustment" score was also computed. The table below presents the results:

	ONE-PARENT Means†	TWO-PARENT Means†	*t*	*p*
Home and Family	17.5	16.8	1.5	>.05
Friends and Peers	19.1	19.4	0.9	>.05
General Behaviors	24.7	25.3	1.1	>.05
Overall Behavioral Adjustment	61.3	61.5	0.7	>.05

†Higher scores reflect *better* adjustment.

Here is how Olsen described her results:

> Contrary to expectations, the behavioral patterns of the children from intact and one-parent homes were very similar. With respect to "Home and Family" behaviors, in fact, children in the one-parent homes were superior. Friendship patterns and interactions with peers were virtually identical in the two groups. In terms of general behaviors, such as crying, pouting, or acting out, the children from the two-parent families showed a slight edge. Overall, the two groups performed about equivalently. Thus, it may be concluded that preschool children who live in one-parent families are not handicapped by the absence of their fathers. Their behaviors are normal and not different from those of their same-aged peers from intact homes. In one area, children from the one-parent home show evidence of more favorable behaviors than those with both parents at home.

1. Review and critique the above description. Suggest alternative ways of describing and interpreting the results. To help you in your critique, here are some guiding questions:

   a. Comment on the content of the excerpt. Did the author omit discussing any important results? Was there any redundancy—could the summary have been more succinct?

   b. Comment on the accuracy of the report. Does the text agree with the table? Does the report imply statistically significant results that were in fact not in the data?

   c. Comment on the style of the report. Does the author use language that is too subjective? Does the author fail to use language that is in keeping with the tentative nature of research? Does the author use jargon or unnecessary technical terms?

    d. Comment on the author's interpretation of the results. Does the author "read too much" into the data? Does the author suggest several possible explanations for the findings? In the interpretation, does the author try to take into consideration such factors as the smallness of the sample, the influence of extraneous variables, inadequacies of the measuring instrument, and so on?

2. Below are several suggested research articles. Skim one (or more) of these articles, focusing especially on the researcher's interpretation of the results. Respond to questions a to d from Exercise D.1 in terms of the actual research study.

- Beckmann, C.A. (1990). Postterm pregnancy: Effects on temperature and glucose regulation. *Nursing Research, 39,* 21-24.
- Kolanowski, A.M. (1990). Restlessness in the elderly: The effect of artificial lighting. *Nursing Research, 39,* 181-183.
- Lu, A.Y., Metzger, B.L., and Therrien, B. (1990). Ethnic differences in physiological responses assosiated with the Valsalva maneuver. *Research in Nursing and Health, 13,* 9-15.
- Rudy, E.B. and Estok, P.J. (1990). Running addiction and dyadic adjustment. *Research in Nursing and Health, 13,* 219-225.
- Young, D.M. and Garvin, B.J. (1990). Nurses' knowledge and attitudes and AIDS patients; perception of confirmation. *Applied Nursing Research, 3,* 105-111.

E. Special Projects

1. Suppose that you were studying maternal behavior in mothers of normal and handicapped children. Fifty mothers from each group are observed interacting with their children (age 7–10) in a laboratory setting for 30 minutes. Some data are presented below:

MEAN NO. OF	MOTHERS WITH NORMAL CHILDREN	MOTHERS WITH HANDICAPPED CHILDREN	*t*
times mother initiates conversations	10.2	12.8	2.3
minutes of silence	14.9	13.8	1.7
times mother laughs or smiles	8.4	7.9	1.2
direct maternal commands	8.7	6.1	3.8
encouraging/supportive comments	4.1	5.7	2.4

Write a brief "results" and "discussion" section for these data.

2. Read the article "Information processing strategies of women enrolled in traditional and nontraditional college majors" by Lois Haggerty, which appeared in the *Western Journal of Nursing Research,* 1990, Vol. 12, pages 525–536. Prepare an abstract for this study.

28
Evaluating Research Reports

Read and critique one or more of the following articles (or other articles in the nursing research literature) and apply the questions in Chapter 28 of the text to the article. Prepare a 2 to 3 page critique summarizing the major strengths and weaknesses of the study.

- Deiriggi, P. M. (1990). Effects of waterbed flotation on indicators of energy expenditure in preterm infants. *Nursing Research*, *39*, 140–147.
- Franks, F. and Faux, S. A. (1990). Depression, stress, mastery, and social resources in four ethnocultural women's groups. *Research in Nursing and Health*, *13*, 283–292.
- Holtzclaw, B. J. (1990). Effects of extremity wraps to control drug-induced shivering: A pilot study. *Nursing Research*, *39*, 280–284.
- Jackson, B. B. (1990). Social support and life satisfaction of black climacteric women. *Western Journal of Nursing Research*, *12*, 9–27.
- Jirovec, M. M. and Wells, T. J. (1990). Urinary incontinence in nursing home residents with dementia. *Applied Nursing Research*, *3*, 112–117.
- Kulig, J. C. (1990). Childbearing beliefs among Cambodian refugee women. *Western Journal of Nursing Research*, *12*, 108–118.
- Lundman, B., Asplund, K., and Norberg, A. (1990). Living with diabetes: Perceptions of well-being. *Research in Nursing and Health*, *13*, 255–262.

- Simpson, T. (1990). and Shaver, J. (1990). Cardiovascular responses to family visits in coronary care unit patients. *Heart and Lung, 19,* 344–351.
- Strumpf, N. E. and Evans, L. K. (1988). Physical restraint of the hospitalized elderly. *Nursing Research, 37,* 132–137.
- Weinbacher, F. M., Littlejohn, C. E. and Conley, P. F. (1990). Growth of bacteria in prefilled syringes stored in home refrigerators. *Applied Nursing Research, 3,* 63–67.

29
Utilization of Nursing Research

A. Matching Exercises

Match each of the strategies from Set B with one of the roles indicated in Set A. Indicate the letter corresponding to your response next to each of the strategies in Set B.

SET A
a. Nursing researchers
b. Nursing faculty/educators
c. Practicing nurses/nursing students
d. Nursing administrators

SET B

1. Become involved in journal club   _____
2. Perform replications   _____
3. Prepare integrative reviews of research literature   _____
4. Offer resources for utilization projects   _____
5. Disseminate findings   _____
6. Specify clinical implications of findings   _____
7. Read research reports critically   _____
8. Foster intellectual curiosity in the work environment   _____
9. Provide a forum for communication between clinicians and researchers   _____
10. Expect evidence that a precedure is effective   _____

B. Completion Exercises

Write the words or phrases that correctly complete the sentences below.

1. _____
   refers to the use of some aspect of a scientific investigation in an application
   unrelated to the original research.

2. There is considerable concern about the _____
   between knowledge production and knowledge utilization.

3. The most well-known nursing research utilization project, conducted in Michigan,
   is the _____ Project.

4. An early regional collaborative utilization project was the _____
   _____ Project.

5. In order for research results to be believable, study findings must be _____
   _____
   in several different settings.

6. The three broad classes of criteria for research utilization are _____
   _____ ,
   clinical relevance, and scientific merit.

7. The issue of_____
   concerns whether it makes sense to implement an innovation in a new practice
   setting.

8. A cost/benefit assessment should consider not only the net cost/gain of implemen-
   tating an innovation but also _____ .

C. Study Questions

1. Define the following terms. Compare your definition with the definition in Chapter 29 of the textbook or in the glossary.

   a. Instrumental utilization: _____
   _____
   _____

   b. Conceptual utilization: _____
   _____
   _____

c. Knowledge creep: _____

_____

_____

d. Decision accretion: _____

_____

_____

e. Awareness stage of adoption: _____

_____

_____

f. Persuasion state of adoption: _____

_____

_____

g. Scientific merit: _____

_____

_____

h. Cost/benefit ratio: _____

_____

_____

2. Prepare an example of a research question that could be posed to improve nursing care in the five phases of the nursing process.
   a. Assessment phase

   b. Diagnosis phase

   c. Planning phase

d. Intervention phase

e. Evaluation phase

3. Think about a nursing procedure about which you have been instructed. What is the basis for this procedure? Determine whether the procedure is based on scientific evidence that the procedure is effective. If it is not based on scientific evidence, on what is it based and why do you think scientific evidence was not used?

4. Identify the factors in your own setting that you think facilitate or inhibit research utilization (or, in an educational setting, the factors that promote or inhibit a climate in which research utilization is valued.)

5. Read Brett's (1987) article regarding the adoption of 14 nursing innovations ("Use of nursing practice research findings," *Nursing Research*, *36*, 344–349) or read a more recent study based on the same 14 innovations by Coyle and Sokop, 1990 ("Innovation adoption behavior among nurses," *Nursing Research*, *39*, 176–180). For each of the 14 innovations, indicate whether you are aware of the findings, persuaded that the findings should be used, use the findings sometimes in a clinical situation, or use the findings always in a clinical situation.

    1.

    2.

    3.

    4.

    5.

    6.

    7.

    8.

9.

10.

11.

12.

13.

14.

6. With regard to the 14 innovations in Brett's study (see Exercise 5 above), select an innovation/finding of which you (or most class members) were unaware. Go to the original source and read the research report. Perform a critique of the study, indicating in particular why you think there may have been barriers to having the innovation implemented in a local setting.

D. *Application Exercise*

1. Below are several suggested research articles. Read one or more of these articles, paying special attention to the Conclusion/Implications section of the report. Evaluate the extent to which you believe the researcher(s)' discussion would facilitate the utilization of the study findings within clinical settings. If possible, suggest some clinical implications that the researchers did not discuss, or discuss the implications in terms of nursing education.

   - Doering, L. and Dracup, K. (1988). Comparisons of cardiac output in supine and lateral positions. *Nursing Research, 37*, 114–118.
   - Harrison, M. J. (1990). A comparison of parental interactions with term and preterm infants. *Research in Nursing and Health, 13*, 173–179.
   - Heidenreich, T. and Giuffre, M. (1990). Postoperative temperature measurement. *Nursing Research, 39*, 153–155.
   - McPhail, A., Pikula, H., Roberts, J., Browne, G. and Harper, D. (1990). Primary nursing: A randomized crossover trial. *Western Journal of Nursing Research, 12*, 188–200.
   - Samples, J. T., Dougherty, M. C., Abrams, R. M. and Batich, C. D. (1988). The dynamic characteristics of circumvaginal muscles. *Journal of Obstetric, Gynecologic, and Neonatal Nursing, 17*, 194–201.

- Therrien, B. (1990). Position modifies carotid artery blood flow velocity during straining. *Research in Nursing and Health, 13*, 69–76.

E. Special Project

1. Select a study from the nursing research literature. Using the utilization criteria indicated in Box 29.1 of the textbook, assess the potential for utilizing the study results in a clinical practice setting. If the study meets the three major classes of criteria for utilization, develop a utilization plan.

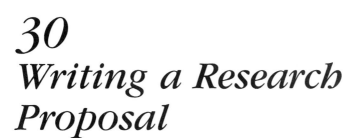

30
Writing a Research Proposal

A. Matching Exercises

Match each statement designating a section of an NIH grant application from Set B with one (or more) of the phrases listed in Set A. Indicate the letter(s) corresponding to your response next to each of the statements in Set B.

SET A
a. Specific Aims section
b. Significance section
c. Preliminary Studies section
d. Experimental Design and Methods section
e. None of these sections

SET B   **RESPONSE**
1. Includes the budget   _____
2. Includes a review of previous research   _____
3. Includes a summary of the study objectives _____
4. Is restricted to three pages   _____
5. Includes a description of the proposed sample _____
6. Has no explicit page limitations   _____
7. Allows the investigators to elaborate on their research
   qualifications   _____

8. Includes rationales for methodological decisions   _____
9. Has a recommended page limitation of 1 page   _____
10. May include the work plan   _____
11. Includes biographical sketches   _____
12. Has a recommended page limitation of 2–3 pages   _____

B. Completion Exercises

1. Proposals often begin with a brief synopsis or _____
   _____ of the proposed research.

2. Objectives stated in the form of _____
   _____ to be tested are generally preferred.

3. The _____
   describes the plan and schedule according to which project tasks would be accomplished.

4. The _____
   translates the project activities into monetary terms.

5. A funding agency often publicizes the _____
   _____
   that will be used in making evaluative decisions about submitted proposals.

6. The person who plays the lead role on a research project is often referred to as
   the _____
   _____ .

7. Applications for research funds through the National Institutes of Health (NIH)
   that are not approved for funding are either _____
   _____ or _____ .

8. The first part of the dual review system within NIH involves a _____
   _____ .

9. Applications that are approved through the Public Health Service are all assigned a
   _____
   _____ .

10. Written critiques of grant applications through the NIH are provided through
    _____ .

11. The two major types of federal disbursements are _____
_____ and _____ .

12. RFP is an acronym for _____
_____ .

C. Study Questions

1. Define the following terms. Compare your definition with the definition in Chapter 30 of the textbook or in the glossary.

   a. Proposal: _____
   _____
   _____

   b. Work plan: _____
   _____
   _____

   c. Gantt chart: _____
   _____
   _____

   d. Application kit: _____
   _____
   _____

   e. R01 Grant: _____
   _____
   _____

   f. AREA award: _____
   _____
   _____

   g. FIRST award: _____
   _____
   _____

h. Priority rating or score: _____

_____

_____

i. Study section: _____

_____

_____

j. Frontmatter: _____

_____

_____

k. RFA: _____

_____

_____

l. Grant: _____

_____

_____

m. Contract: _____

_____

_____

2. Chapter 30 of the text described several major sections of Public Health Service grant applications. In which sections would the following statements ordinarily be found?

a. The third task, the screening of volunteers for eligibility and the assignment of subjects to experimental and control groups, will be accomplished in the fourth week of the project and will require five person-days of effort.

_____

_____

b. The primary hypothesis is that paraplegics who receive pool therapy will perform better on tests of muscle strength than those who receive other types of exercise.

_____

_____

c. Dr. Treas, who will direct the proposed research, has recently completed a three-year longitudinal study of the coping mechanisms of parents with a Down's syndrome infant.

d. The major threat to the internal validity of the proposed study is selection bias, which will be dealt with through the careful selection of comparison subjects and through statistical adjustment of pre-existing differences.

e. All subjects will be asked to sign informed consent forms.

f. The proposed research will have the potential of restructuring the delivery of health care in rural areas.

D. Application Exercises

Below is a "Specific Aims" section from a grant application that was funded by the U.S. Office of Adolescent Pregnancy Programs.* This application is also referred to in Chapter 30 of the text.

A. SPECIFIC AIMS

Substantial percentages of children in our society are born to young women who are teenagers. Despite the growth of interest in the "epidemic" of teenage pregnancy, relatively little attention has been paid to the parenting styles and behaviors of young mothers or to the development of their children, particularly in well-designed, longitudinal research.

    The proposed research will use a combined observational/interview approach to collect information about the parental styles and attitudes, the family and home environment, and children's development in a sample of about 300 low-income young women who first became pregnant when they were 17 or

*D. Polit, "Parenting among low-income teenage mothers," awarded to Humanalysis, Inc., 1985. Reprinted with permission of Humanalysis, Inc.

younger, and whose oldest child is now about 5 years of age. Three rounds of interviews with these mothers have already been completed, in which extensive information about their backgrounds, economic circumstances, social support networks, household structure, psychological characteristics, and use of formal services (including parenting education) was gathered. The baseline interviews with these women, conducted either during their pregnancy or shortly after delivery, also measured parenting knowledge and perceived competence in parenting skills. The women in the sample reside in six geographically dispersed communities (Bedford-Stuyvesant, NY; Harlem, NY; Phoenix, AZ; San Antonio, TX; Riverside, CA; and Fresno, CA) and represent an ethnic mix of black, Hispanic, and white young mothers.

The longitudinal nature of this research will make it possible to test a comprehensive model of the effects of maternal age on several parenting and child development outcomes. The availability of extensive background information will also permit background influences (such as pre-delivery family structure and financial circumstances, early school experiences, educational aspirations, self-esteem, and family size expectations) to be controlled, yielding a more sensitive test of the hypothesized effects. In brief, the proposed research will examine the extent to which a teen mother's parenting knowledge is influenced by her age at first birth and her exposure to parenting education classes, net of other factors. Parenting behaviors (such as warmth, punitiveness, and stimulation of the child's learning) are hypothesized to be influenced by three major factors: characteristics of the mother (including her parenting knowledge), characteristics of the child, and contextual factors such as stress and social support. Finally, the model predicts that child development outcomes (including cognitive development, social/behavioral adjustment, and physical health) are a function of parenting behaviors and the home environment, as well as characteristics of the child.

1. Review and critique this section of the grant application. To assist you in your critique, here are some guiding questions:

   a. Is the presentation sufficiently specific? Does the author make overly general statements about what the research will accomplish?

   b. Is the presentation clear and succinct? Is it direct and to the point?

   c. Does the presentation sound convincing and authoritative? Does the researcher seem knowledgeable about the substantive issues?

   d. Do the objectives sound manageable? That is, does it appear that the researcher will actually be able to accomplish her objectives, or is the scope of her objectives overly broad?

2. A nurse researcher wanted to study student attrition among minority nursing school students.* She proposed a critical incidents study of the experiences leading to minority students' decisions to drop out of their nursing programs. The study was to involve interviews with 150 minority dropouts in three states. Below is a tentative budget for such a project.

BUDGET-MINORITY ATTRITION STUDY

Personnel		
Rodgers (Principal Investigator)	40 wks @ 800/wk	$32,000
Campbell (Interviewer)	10 wks @ 400/wk	4,000
Wolfe (Interviewer)	10 wks @ 400/wk	4,000
Kulka (Research Assistant)	16 wks @ 275/wk	4,400
Cherlin (Admin. Assistant)	26 wks @ 325/wk	8,450
		$52,850
+ Fringe Benefits (25%)		13,213
TOTAL PERSONNEL		$66,063
Nonpersonnel		
Supplies 50/mo. × 12 mos.		$ 600
Xeroxing 50/mo. × 12 mos.		600
Printing Instruments		500
Data entry 300 records × .50/record		150
Travel 3000 miles × 0.25/mile		750
Consultants 10 days @ 250/day		2,500
TOTAL NONPERSONNEL		$ 5,100
TOTAL DIRECT COSTS		**$71,163**

Review and comment on this budget in terms of the following:

a. The inclusion of all relevant budget categories for the proposed study

b. Your perceptions of whether any given category is over- or underbudgeted.

E. Special Projects

1. Prepare a one-page "Special Aims" section for a research project you would like to conduct.

2. Identify at least one federal agency and two foundations that might be appropriate for sending a research proposal for a project in which you are interested.

---

*This example is fictitious.